Limiting dilution analysis of cells of the immune system

Limiting dilution analysis of cells of the immune system

SECOND EDITION

IVAN LEFKOVITS
Basel Institute for Immunology

HERMAN WALDMANN
Sir William Dunn School of Pathology, University of Oxford

with
LDA SOFTWARE
developed by
P. Rovensky, J. Rubes and T. Beran

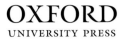
OXFORD
UNIVERSITY PRESS

OXFORD

UNIVERSITY PRESS

Great Clarendon Street, Oxford OX2 6DP

Oxford University Press is a department of the University of Oxford
and furthers the University's aim of excellence in research, scholarship,
and education by publishing worldwide in

Oxford New York

Athens Auckland Bangkok Bogotá Buenos Aires Calcutta
Cape Town Chennai Dar es Salaam Delhi Florence Hong Kong Istanbul
Karachi Kuala Lumpur Madrid Melbourne Mexico City Mumbai
Nairobi Paris São Paulo Singapore Taipei Tokyo Toronto Warsaw

and associated companies in Berlin Ibadan

Oxford is a trade mark of Oxford University Press

Published in the United States
by Oxford University Press Inc., New York

First edition published 1979

© Cambridge University Press

Second edition published 1999

© Ivan Lefkovits and Herman Waldmann, 1999

Software © P. Rovensky, J. Rubes, and T. Beran, 1999

The moral rights of the author have been asserted

British Library Cataloguing in Publication Data

Data available

Library of Congress Cataloging- in-Publication Data
Lefkovits, Ivan.
Limiting dilution analysis of cells of the immune system/Ivan
Lefkovits, Hermann Waldmann; with LDA software developed by P.
Rovensky, J. Rubes, and T. Beran, — 2nd ed.

Includes bibliographical references and index.
1. Lymphocytes — Research — Methodology. 2. Plaque assay technique.
3. Immunology — Statistical methods. 4. Dilution. I. Waldmann,
Herman. II. Title.
[DNLM: 1. B-Lymphocytes — chemistry. 2. Indicator Dilution
Techniques. 3. B-Lymphocytes — immunology. 4. T-Lymphocytes —
chemistry. 5. T-Lymphocytes — immunology. 6. Immunity, Cellular.
WH 200 L493L 1999]
QR185.8.L9L43 1999 616.07'9 — dc21 98-50046

ISBN 0 19 850128 5 (Hbk)

Typeset by EXPO Holdings, Malaysia
Printed in Great Britain
on acid-free paper by
Redwood Books Ltd, Trowbridge, Wilts

Contents

Refer to http://www.path.ox.ac.uk/lda/
for

- Further information on the software
- Software updates
- News on media and instrumentation
- Additional references
- Reader's comments
- Information about the authors

Orders and information about related books may also be accessed via this site
or on http://www.oup.co.uk/isbn0-19-850128-5/.

Preface

This monograph is the revised version of a book which was first assembled 20 years ago. The period between these two editions has witnessed some revolutionary changes in cell and molecular biology: not only have these had a substantive impact on the theoretical foundations of immunology but they have also greatly amplified the methodological armaments which are available to study function.

Why then should a method that was so useful 20 years ago remain one of choice in the modern era? There are two reasons. First, this method has evolved from its previous role as a basic laboratory tool to one applicable to many different disciplines and to clinical application. Second, the new methodologies (such as PCR) can complement the old, so that single-cell assays, or assays of subcellular particles such as viruses, are now more amenable to the limiting dilution approach.

The above arguments, combined with the fact that the first edition of the LDA monograph is out-of-print, provided the impetus to prepare a new edition of the book. A further incentive was the exciting prospect of incorporating an extensive software package for LDA analysis and simulation.

Although the book includes many new features, the overall scheme remains the same as in the first edition. We have retained the same title for historical reasons, although it might have been opportune to add a subtitle to indicate that the methodology can also be applied to cells other than those of the immune system. We wrote the first edition primarily for immunologists, but we have expanded this edition so that it will be useful in other fields of research where PCR methodology is used to analyse rare cells (cancer cells, cells expressing rare mutations, etc.).

We anticipate that this volume will prove to be useful, additional reading for students of biology and medicine who feel that the standard textbooks cover the application of Poisson distribution superficially.

We will update the LDA program and the simulation software at regular intervals in the future and we hope that supplementary subprograms will be developed. We intend to make these updates available on the Web.

Ivan Lefkovits
Herman Waldmann

Acknowledgements

During the preparation of this manuscript I obtained some insight into the working of Oxford University Press. Interactions with Drs Stuart McRobbie, Melissa Levitt and Beth Knight contributed to the smooth transition of the project to its final palpable form of a manuscript. I was impressed by the ingenuity of Claire Walker and Jonathan Coleclough of the art department with whom I had contact over the preparation of the book cover. It was a great pleasure for me to work with Phil Longford on the figures and computer-aided images. All in all, the atmosphere at OUP was so pleasant that that in itself would be an incentive to write another book.

The manuscript was typed and compiled by Leslie Nicklin, editorial assistant. She dealt with the many drafts, the many finals, and the many final-finals, during the preparatory stages, then via email and fax during my sabbatical in Oxford, and finally over long, weary hours on the final stages after I was back in Basel. Her calm and wise approach helped to offset the hectic, sometimes critical, periods. Randy Baron solved many of the computer-related problems, and Bert Temminck supervised the installation of the LDA and simulation programs. Hans-Peter Stahlberger provided the non-computer artwork. He had done it for the first edition and again he produced those figures which are in the same style as the original ones. With great skill Catherine Forbes finalised many of the computer-aided figures. Bea Pfeiffer prepared photographs of the microcultures trays depicted in the Appendix.

A special thanks goes to Dr Mauro Buser. His constructive suggestions helped finalise the chapter on statistics. He contributed both with some basic concepts concerning the confidence limits of the slope and with the fine details on the chi-squared test. This help was very timely seeing as my colleague and friend, Charley Steinberg – who was always around when I needed to discuss a scientific issue with him – retired just when the draft manuscript was complete.

A considerable portion of the book was written during my sabbatical at the Sir William Dunn School of Pathology in Oxford. I am indebted to my host and co-author of this book, Herman Waldmann, for creating a wonderful and stimulating atmosphere for my visit. I also received valuable support from Drs Paul Fairchild and Steve Cobbold. Computer officer John Marriott helped during my entire sabbatical and his assistance will continue after publication when he will probably take care of the website.

Finally, while in Oxford I enjoyed the hospitality of Lincoln College. Elected a member of the SCR, I used the dining rights extensively. The vintage port available from the college wine cellar provided the requisite inspiration for the many hours of work on this monograph.

Ivan Lefkovits

To be frank, I hate writing anything larger than a conventional scientific paper, and even that often drives me to despair. I recall that the first edition of this book was tough enough. In those days we had no word processors, and everything needed to be written by hand a few times, before we could pass drafts onto our secretaries. These days we have word processors, fax machines and email attachments. So when Ivan suggested we do a second edition you might think I would jump at the opportunity. Fortunately, I had started a new job in Oxford, and so I thought I could justify to Ivan why it might not be such a good idea. His reaction was sympathetic, making me feel even more guilty. He maintained a dignified silence, and I thought the whole idea was now dead.

Then came the notion of his coming to the Dunn School of Pathology. What a great idea to have my good friend nearby. I knew everyone would enjoy his presence (and indeed they did!). He had a nice house near the laboratory; was able to walk across the park, and you would have thought this was the opportunity for him to relax. To my horror, on the day he arrived in the laboratory he indicated that now he could see just what I did in my new job, and could ensure that the chapter writing could take place in small windows of opportunity. He did a great deal in the time, and I tried to respond, although subconsciously I was trying to find more avoidance distractions. I started raising money for new buildings, so that my table could seem full of papers, architects' drawings, spreadsheets, etc. No room to write about LDA!

Well that didn't deter Ivan – when he returned to Basel he invited me to the Institute on my way back from a scientific meeting. From the moment I arrived in his Institute he declared that he was going to stay with me day and night; till the book was finished. I had no choice. I know that Ivan's wife Hana must have felt he was being cruel, but Ivan recognised that he needed to be cruel to be kind. Anyway we did it. The final evening was as you might expect a splendid one with a wonderful dinner with Hana and Ivan, and Ivan behaving as if all of this had been the norm.

Ivan is a very experienced author and editor. There is no doubt in my mind that I would not have co-authored a book with anyone else in this period of my life. His tenacity, gentleness and diplomacy left me no choice. In the end though I felt a great sense of satisfaction. We have a good book, and he is still a great friend! Even better, the Dunn School has two new buildings!

Finally, many of you will have read articles saying that LDA of T-cell function is passé because of the emergence of the tetramer technology that counts antigen-binding T cells. Please remember that the information you get from tetramers is not the same as what you get from LDA. Counting antigen-binding cells will not tell you how many are involved in function, and so functional assays will continue to be important.

I hope that I have given you some insight into the style of my senior author. On a more serious note, Ivan, of course, pioneered LDA in immunology. He has always been enormously generous with his know-how, and I was very lucky as a graduate student to be given the opportunity to work with, and to learn from, him. That has been one of my real pleasures in science.

Herman Waldmann

Software development

The software presented in this book was written and assembled by Pavol Rovensky, Jan Rubes and Tomas Beran. It was prepared and tested in several instalments.

The early steps in developing this program were initiated in 1993 when Pavol Rovensky spent a few months in my laboratory in Basel developing a software package for data management in a two-dimensional gel electrophoresis laboratory. He read the Limiting Dilution Monograph, and when he realised that I was toying with the idea of assembling a new edition he offered to write a program for evaluating limiting dilution data. Then when he found out that I use simulation tools when teaching immunology courses at Philipps University in Marburg and elsewhere, he suggested writing two independent pieces of software, one for evaluating LDA data and the other for LDA simulation. At that time, i.e. when he wrote the first 'fragment' of the software, he was still studying medicine in Prague. In the meantime, not only has he attained his MD degree, but at the time of writing he is about to complete his studies in computer science at the Technical University of Prague.

Pavol Rovensky and I went through my notes and prepared the backbone for both software packages. From that moment onwards he worked independently, partly in Prague and during several visits to Basel in 1995 and 1996. He teamed-up with Jan Rubes, a graduate of the Technical University of Prague, and, for the last stages of the program development, with Tomas Beran, a young programmer from Prague. It was therefore a veritable Czech team, working mostly in Prague, though for the final 'push' they joined me in Oxford where I spent my sabbatical in 1997.

The software is as complete as we could achieve with the means available - time being the most precious commodity. Although this software - as part of the book - is a definitive 'product', we will use the Internet to add further features to it.

I wish to express my grateful thanks to all three members of the team. Without their input this LDA book would be but a skeleton.

Ivan Lefkovits

On my first visit to Ivan Lefkovits' laboratory I received the impression that although the methodology of two-dimensional gel electrophoresis and cDNA libraries were involved in the day-to-day experiments, the underlying interest of the group was in 'quantitative cellular immunology'. The term 'limiting dilution analysis' was new to me and I knew very little about how to apply Poisson distribution to cell biology. My early discussions with Ivan concentrated on examples of Poissonian events (many of them given in this book), then they focused on experiments applying cell cultures, and finally we put down on paper the first outline of the prospective software.

Ivan's enthusiastic reaction to the first software version was a real incentive for me to continue. However, the project turned out to be more encompassing than he had intended and more complex than I had imagined. But still, Ivan's drive to move along whenever a new (and better and more complex) version became available, and his trust that the project would eventually be completed, were highly motivating factors. In fact, the LDA project became a crucial turning point for me as it led to my decision to dedicate almost all my future work to developing software technology. Thus, I thank Ivan for his continuous guidance and for his help whenever problems – small or large – had to be resolved.

I am especially indebted to Bert Temminck of the Basel Institute for Immunology who directed my first steps in the field of computers and software. Bert always found time to share his knowledge of system management with me and he helped me to devise the method required to implement the LDA software. Indeed, it was Bert who made me realise that the final 'product' could only be achieved if I assembled a semi-professional team to help with it. I succeeded in doing this and thus had the pleasure to work with Jan Rubes and Tomas Beran on the project (and in parallel on some others). I wish to thank them for the creativity they showed during each stage of the work.

I also wish to thank Vladimir Radovansky and Tomas Mohelsky who were always around when I needed reliable advice.

I would like to take this opportunity to thank my parents who, as always, gave me immense support throughout my work on the project.

My gratitude also goes to Knoll Pharmaceuticals for my personal grant which enabled me to devote a great deal of time to the project without undergoing any financial strain.

In every respect it was a rewarding experience for me and it may prove to be a stepping stone for designing further interesting schemes. Hopefully the reactions of the users of the LDA software will provide an impetus for assembling an even better and even more sophisticated version of the LDA software.

Pavol Rovensky

The Basel Institute for Immunology was founded and is supported by F. Hoffmann-La Roche Ltd., Basel, Switzerland

Abbreviations and meanings of Latin and Greek letters

Abbreviations

ATxBM	Adult thymectomised irradiated bone marrow reconstituted
BMT	Bone marrow transplant
BSS	Balanced salt solution
CD4	Markers on T cells
CD8	Markers on T cells
Con A	Concanavalin A
CTL	Cytotoxic T lymphocytes
DRBC	Donkey erythrocytes
EBV-LPD	Epstein–Barr virus-induced lymphoproliferative disease
FGG	Fowl gamma globulin
GVHD	Graft versus host disease
GVL	Graft versus leukaemia
HIV	Human immunodeficiency virus
HRBC	Horse erythrocytes
IFN-γ	Interferon gamma
IL-2	Interleukin-2
KLH	Keyhole limpet haemocyanin
LPC	Limiting precursor cells
LPS	Lipopolysaccharide
MEM	Minimal essential medium
MHC	Major histocompatibility complex
MLR	Mixed lymphocyte reaction
NIP	4-hydroxy-5-iodo-3-nitrophenylacetyl
OA or OVA	Ovalbumin
PBS	Phosphate-buffered saline
PCR	Polymerase chain reaction
PFC	Plaque-forming cells
PPD	Purified protein derivative
RPMI	Culture medium
SRBC	Sheep erythrocytes
Th1 cells	T-helper cells type 1
Th2 cells	T-helper cells type 2
TI	Thymus independent
TNP	Trinitrophenyl
Ts cells	T-suppressor cells

Listed below are the Latin and Greek letters used in this book with their meanings:

a	slope, also value in 2 x 2 table see b, c, d
b	value in 2 x 2 table see a, c, d
c	number of cells, value in 2 x 2 tables
$\bar{c}$	average clone size
d	value in 2 x 2 table see a, b, c
df	degree of freedom
e	constant (approx. 2.71828)
F	fraction
F_0	fraction of nonresponding cultures
$\hat{F}_0$	expected value of F_0
f	frequency
k	number of assay plates
m	number of cells in the target theory, see also n
n	number of cells, in another context number of clones, number of cells in the hit theory, number of samples, see also m
P	probability
p	probability of success
q	probability of failure
R	ratio
r	number of cells (integers 0, 1, 2, 3 . . .)
t	t-test (Student's t-test)
V	variance
w_-	number of nonresponding cultures
$\hat{w}_-$	expected value of w_-
w_R	number of responding cultures
$\hat{w}_R$	expected value of w_R
w_T	total number of cultures
x	random variable
$\bar{x}$	sample mean
α	tail area (probability)
χ^2	chi-squared
Δ	difference (from delta)
μ	mean
Σ	sum
σ	standard deviation
σ^2	variance

1   Introduction

1.1   The immune response

The field of immunology has been one of the most rapidly advancing branches
of cell biology for a variety of reasons. The most significant is that the activity
of a single lymphocyte can be easily measured through its products, whether
they be antibodies, cytokines or other molecules that lyse target cells. An
added advantage is that immunologically relevant cells, whether present in the
circulation or in lymphoid organs, do not bear long-term physical associations
with any organ, or even each other. It has therefore been easy to isolate cell
populations and to follow the fates of single cells and their progeny. The ease
with which most lymphocyte functions have lent themselves to *in vitro* representation, has enabled sophisticated quantitation to be applied to the processes
of cell growth, differentiation and function.

   The immune system of a human may comprise say 10^{12} lymphocytes. The
capacity to recognise and react to the universe of antigens is confined within
this number. Each lymphocyte is restricted in the diversity of receptors it
expresses so that in the case of B cells only one molecular species is expressed,
and in the case of T cells one, but at the most two. The way in which T cells and
B cells do this is beyond the scope of this monograph, but suffice it to say that
the requirement that the immune system recognise discrete sets of antigens
from the outside world is endowed to clones of cells, which remain available
after self-tolerance processes have purged or silenced any potential autoreactive members.

   An immune response begins when lymphocytes which are 'precommitted'
to a particular receptor engage antigen. The events that follow involve clonal
proliferation, differentiation and death of many progeny cells. Classical cellular
immunology has largely been concerned with the events at the beginning (for
example antigen dose, quality, context) and at the end (quality and quantity of
response) with very little information gained on the intermediate events.
Information on the events in this 'ecliptic' period has largely been extrapolated
from experiments that involve simple perturbations of the system with defined
probes. Information on the numbers of participating clones, on the clone size,
the interactions of clones with each other, and the proportion of clonal

members which could differentiate, was simply unavailable through traditional experimental approaches.

In the early 1970s, the introduction of lymphocyte *in vitro* culture systems provided the opportunity to focus in more depth on the clonal aspects of immunity. One of the first issues that could be addressed was that of frequencies of B cells and T cells precommitted to respond to any given antigen. Those early experiments led for the first time to the development of a whole series of approaches dependent on 'Limiting Dilution Analysis' (LDA) that examined how individual antigen-specific lymphocytes, anonymous within the larger population of lymphocytes, might interact with other antigen-specific cells; how they responded to growth factors; how they might be regulated; and indeed how they might be inactivated or tolerised.

1.2   Cells of the immune system

Much of our knowledge of the immune system has come from defining the cell types and interactions involved in the immune responses required to eliminate pathogens. This has led to a description of subsets of T cells, B cells and a range of accessory cells that participate. Historically the process started with definition of function, for example, T cells helping B cells make antibody, from which the concept of T-helper cells arose. Current dogma defines 'help' as coming in two forms, mediated by so-called Th1 and Th2-type helper cells, both included within the CD4 T-cell subset. Similarly, killer activity within T cells has been explained primarily through the description of cytotoxic T cells (CTLs) included within the CD8 T-cell subset. Recently, however, it has become clear that the capacity to kill other cells can be elicited by many cell types, even T-helper cells, through the expression of particular cell-surface molecules with a physiological role in limiting the growth of other cell types. The message is that individual cells may take on a variety of functions under particular circumstances, and that all readouts of such functions are operational.

If we think about more subtle functions of cells in the immune system, then the reader should understand that many immune phenomena may not be represented with as slick a title as the 'T-helper cell'. For example, there are numerous descriptions of T cells that suppress an immune function. Yet without consensus very few workers are prepared to use the term 'T-suppressor cell'. Indeed, mistakes and misfortunes of the past have discouraged use of this term. The lack of useful nomenclature for cells with regulatory functions creates real difficulties in scientific communication, and almost certainly limits research activity in this area. For our purposes, in trying to devise ways to measure cells with 'downregulatory' functions, we need to adopt a suitable nomenclature. For that reason, in this monograph we will use the generic term Ts (or T-suppressor cell).

If we accept the notion that the frequency of cells performing a particular function in a defined context can be measured, then the LDA approach can be used to quantitate the activities of all lymphocyte, dendritic cell and accessory cell populations in responses which measure both upregulatory or downregulatory functions.

1.3   Why should one use a functional approach to study the immune system?

'If you cannot study function study structure'

In his summary to the Cold Spring Harbor Symposia in 1967 Niels Kaj Jerne pointed out the dichotomy of studying structure and function of the immune system: '...if you cannot study function, study structure' (Jerne, 1967). The truth is what one studies often reflects the technologies available at the time. If we look back at the research tools available in immunology in this century we can identify three distinct waves of methodological advance.

The development of immunochemical methods

Since immunoglobulin is the most abundant molecular species (apart from albumin) in the circulation of animals, it is perhaps not surprising that the methodology for assaying these molecules developed first.

Advances in cellular immunological methods

The analysis of cells playing a role in the immune system has a curious history. Prior to the postulation of the natural selection and clonal selection theories for the immune system (Jerne, 1955; Burnet, 1957), there was no basis for searching and identifying cells involved in the immune response. As long as antibody was thought of as a single molecular species that could adapt and adjust to any antigen, then there was no incentive to search for a cellular basis. Only after Burnet (1957) postulated 1 cell = 1 antibody, and after Gowans (1963) showed that it was the lymphocyte which represented the basic functional unit of the immune system, did the revolution in the methodology of cellular assays become possible. Jerne's method for identifying single antibody-producing cells (1963), and Mishell and Dutton's method for inducing primary immune responses with mouse spleen cells (1967) were the crucial components on which the basis for modern cellular immunology was laid.

Revolution in molecular biology methods

The development of methods by which stretches of genes were cut and ligated at will, and by which the molecules could be amplified to any desired copy number by the polymerase chain reaction, produced a massive shift of emphasis in biological research. It suddenly became considerably easier to study genes (i.e. structure) than gene products (i.e. function).

Maybe Jerne's statement '... if you cannot study function, study structure' could be paraphrased to 'if you cannot study the activity of a molecule, study the gene coding for it'. However, life isn't really that simple. We often need knowledge of the function to study the structure, and often structural information leads to new discoveries of function. The two are irrevocably intertwined. This is true also of the methods in immunochemistry, cellular immunology and molecular biology. We need them all despite the apparent imbalances in their utility. After all, some methods were developed to perfection and then superseded by new ones, while others survived and have stood the test of time.

1.4   Applications in medicine

The LDA approach to enumerating immunologically relevant cells, has established itself with a value well beyond that of an experimental tool for understanding how the immune system works. It is now commonplace in the arena of allogeneic transplantation, especially of bone marrow, for laboratories to calculate the frequency of reactive cells (donor vs. host and vice versa) to establish the likelihood of a good tissue match. It is indeed refreshing to hear clinicians talking about precursor frequencies of helper and cytotoxic T cells as if they were simple and obvious parameters, no different to standards such as haemoglobin, red cell count, electrolytes and so on. What has made this so attractive to investigators is the realisation that a measure that purports to represent the total response is really the integral or the residue of all the previous events that took place with no history of the biological warfare (the life and death of population members) that had given rise to it. The precursor frequency, by its nature, largely represents what was there at the start, and has merely been exposed by the experimenter. It has a sense of solidity about it, and we are not surprised at how the clinical community have embraced it.

1.5   Beyond immunology

There is nothing special about LDA that should limit its use just to analysis of cells of the immune system. Any cell population whose members can be isolated as single cell suspensions, and whose functions can be measured *in vitro*, should be amenable to similar analytical approaches. For example, the analyses of precursor frequencies and clone sizes should be applicable to haematopoiesis, the biology of neoplastic cells and their response to chemotherapeutic agents. As the technologies for studying stem cell biology in the growth and modelling of solid organs improve, then so will the need for LDA to enable one to isolate stem cell-dependent events from those of more differentiated cell types. Even though the biology of other cellular systems will probably be less complex than that of the very flexible immune system, many of the ways we use LDA in the latter should be applicable to the former.

The secret to LDA is to be able to amplify the clonal products of individual cells so as to confidently score the presence or absence of a precursor. Once one can do that then LDA can be applied to any randomly distributing cellular or subcellular system you wish to analyse. The amplification mechanisms could be natural consequences of the activity of the particle which is distributing or they could be 'artificially' contrived so as to score an event where natural mechanisms are not available.

2 From Poisson to Schrödinger

In some scientific disciplines a reference to the past can be tedious and dull, while in others it deepens our understanding of the issue under scrutiny. The history behind Poisson distribution is fascinating. It bears witness to the social and political aspects of society (*probabilité des jugements en matière criminelle*), shows the versatility of the concept (physics, biology) and last but not least shows that a good experiment performed 120 years ago is for today's reader as interesting as a good experiment described in the latest issue of *Science* or *Nature*.

2.1 Poisson's jury

RECHERCHES

SUR LA

PROBABILITÉ DES JUGEMENTS

EN MATIÈRE CRIMINELLE

ET EN MATIÈRE CIVILE,

PRÉCÉDÉES

DES RÈGLES GÉNÉRALES DU CALCUL DES PROBABILITÉS;

PAR S.-D. POISSON,

Membre de l'Institut et du Bureau des Longitudes de France; des Sociétés Royales de Londres et d'Édimbourg; des Académies de Berlin, de Stockholm, de Saint-Pétersbourg, d'Upsal, de Boston, de Turin, de Naples, etc.; des Sociétés, italienne, astronomique de Londres, Philomatique de Paris, etc.

Poisson, in his treatise *Recherches sur la Probabilité des Jugements* (Paris 1837), develops a probability distribution which in its original version has the following form:

$$P = \left(1 + \omega + \frac{\omega^2}{1.2} + \frac{\omega^3}{1.2.3} + \dots + \frac{\omega^n}{1.2.3\dots n} \right) e^{-\omega},$$

pour la probabilité qu'un événement dont la chance à chaque épreuve est la fraction très petite $\frac{\omega}{\mu}$, n'arrivera pas plus de n fois dans un très grand nombre μ d'épreuves.

Poisson's intention was to examine the optimum jury size in order to assure a fair outcome to a trial, in spite of the chance that some jury members vote erroneously. It is said that the 12-member jury dates from Poisson's time.

The book by Poisson reveals that the distribution which he derived was not yet called 'Poisson distribution' since obviously the author would not have made a self-reference.

2.2   Lister's study on the nature of fermentation

When making his first appearance as a teacher at King's College London, Joseph Lister delivered a lecture in which he described experiments on lactic fermentation (Lister, 1878). They dealt with the inoculation of numerous aliquots of milk samples with graded numbers of lactic bacteria. It is apparent that Lister was not acquainted with the mathematical armament of Poisson distribution nor did he provide a calculation model. But still, in our view he devised the first limiting dilution experiment.

Lister explains in his lecture:

'If you get milk from a dairy and keep it long enough, it is certain to turn sour and curdle, then, after a while, there comes a certain mould upon the surface, the *Oïdium lactis*, which constitutes the sort of bloom there is upon a cream cheese;'

And he continues:

'you may be tempted to suppose that these were changes to which the milk was disposed from its own inherent properties as it comes from the cow's udder. '

He describes the first part of the experiment:

'It had been a drizzly morning, and I might fairly hope that some of the multitudes of organisms existing in the little orchard might have been washed down and that the air might thus have been somewhat purified... I got the dairywoman to milk the cow without drawing the hand over the teat, performing the operation by an action of the fingers in succession, so that the end of the teat should always be exposed. Her hands were washed with water, and the cow's udder also, and she having squirted out a little milk to wash away any organisms from the orifice of the duct, the glass cap which protected the larger tube from dust was removed and the end of the tube was held in the immediate vicinity of the teat; a few drachms were introduced, then the cap was readjusted, and then these little glasses were filled by the simple expedient of alternately relaxing and compressing with the finger and thumb on the caoutchouc, so that there was as little disturbance as possible of the organisms that might be supposed to be introduced in spite of my care.'

As expected, some of the samples remained pure, others underwent fermentation. The 'pure' samples tasted sweet, they fulfilled all the criteria of fresh milk. The experiment gave an 'all or none' response, but the crucial part of the assay, one which makes it a true limiting dilution, is as follows:

'It occurred to me that if we could estimate with some degree of accuracy the number of bacteria present in a given quantity of souring milk, and then if we were to dilute the milk with a proportionate quantity of boiled water, we might have the diluted milk so arranged that every drop with which we should inoculate boiled milk might contain, on the average, one bacterium; and if we should do so, as it would be practically certain that the bacteria would not be distributed with absolute uniformity, we should expect that we might have, as the result of these various inoculations, some glasses with the lactic fermentation, some glasses without it, some with the *Bacterium lactis*, and some without it;...I found that it was needful to add no less than one million parts of boiled water to the milk to ensure that there should be rather less than one bacterium, on the average, to every drop. Then with drops of that size I inoculated five glasses of boiled milk, and the result was that out of the five only one curdled; but one did curdle and soured, and that one had the *Bacterium lactis* in abundance; the others did not curdle, underwent no fermentation whatsoever, and had no bacteria in them...These five covered test-tubes which you see before you, containing boiled milk in their lower part, were inoculated each with a drop calculated to contain two bacteria; these other five similar test-tubes were inoculated each with a drop calculated to contain one bacterium; these five liqueur glasses were also inoculated with drops each calculated to contain one bacterium; and one other liqueur glass with a drop calculated to contain four bacteria. The result was that the specimen with the drop calculated to contain four bacteria soured and curdled in a few days; and all these five calculated to have two bacteria to a drop curdled also in a few days. The milk, you see, is perfectly solid...I will now deprive this one of the protection in which it has hitherto lived. [Professor Lister, having removed the glass shade and glass cap from one of the liqueur glasses, proceeded to drink part of its contained milk.] It is perfectly sweet. It has a slight flavour of suet, which M. Pasteur has described as resulting from the oxidation of the oleaginous material of the milk. If any gentleman likes to taste it after the lecture, he can do so.'

2.3   Horse-kicks in the Prussian army

A famous example of events distributed in the Poisson series is the collection of Bortkewitsch's data (1898) from the Prussian Army Corps on the number of people killed by horse-kicks. Records of ten army corps for twenty years correspond to 20 x 10 = 200 corps-years. Obviously the chance of a man being killed by a horse-kick on any one day is exceedingly small, but since the number of people in the corps was large and they were exposed to the risk for a whole year, some lethal accidents usually occurred, and the numbers conformed to the Poisson distribution.

Total number of men killed	122
Number of observations (corps-years)	200
Mean number of men killed per corps-year	$\mu = 0.61$

Table 2.1. The number of people in the Prussian army killed by horse-kicks

Frequency distribution		Number of corps-years with N deaths	
N	F_N	Expected	Observed
0	0.543	108.7	109
1	0.331	66.3	65 (65)
2	0.101	20.2	22 (22x2)
3	0.021	4.1	3 (3x3)
4	0.003	0.6	1 (1x4)
5	0.0004	0.1	0
6	0	0	0
	0.999	200	200 (122)

The above table indicates that the findings of 1, 2, 3 and 4 death fits very well with the Poissonian expectation. The reader is advised to re-read the arguments and inspect the table again once he gets acquainted with sections 3.5 and 3.6.

2.4   Student

In 1907, seventy years after the original publication of Poisson's probability distribution, Gossett (who published under the pseudonym 'Student') arrived at the Poisson series when considering theoretical frequencies in yeast cell samples or erythrocyte samples counted in a haemocytometer. In Student's publication the distribution is derived in a very simple manner as a limit of the binomial distribution. Apparently Student was not aware of Poisson's work.

2.5   Rutherford and Geiger

The Poisson distribution was also brilliantly applied by Rutherford and Geiger (1910) in a work on probability variation in the distribution of α particles. Poisson is not mentioned in this work either, but the distribution is derived by Bateman (1910) in an addendum to Rutherford and Geiger's paper.

2.6   Bell System Technical Journal

Interesting examples of frequency distributions, to which the Poisson distribution is a fairly good approximation, are given in a number of papers in the *Bell System Technical Journal* (Campbell, 1923; Molina and Crowell, 1924; Thorndike, 1926). Those readers who are interested in the historical aspects of statistical methods, and especially those who have access to a good library, should browse through *Biometrika*, a journal founded by Karl Pearson. It is remarkable that on the one hand Student published his famous paper 'The probable error of a mean' in *Biometrika*, while on the other hand several statisticians refused to publish in *Biometrika* because of personal conflict and disagreements with Pearson.

Some relevant papers from *Biometrika* are listed in the references ('Student', 1908; Fisher, 1915; Pearson, 1924, 1939; Clopper and Pearson, 1934; Welch, 1937; Gordon, 1939; Haldane, 1939; Neyman, 1941).

We also recommend a fine – 80 pages long – paper on various aspects of biological samplings by Eisenhart and Wilson (1943).

2.7   Hits of flying bombs on London

During the flying-bomb attacks on London by German V2 rockets in World War II, it was frequently believed that the bomb-hits tended to be grouped in clusters. After the war, Clarke (1946) analysed all recorded hits. He selected a relevant area, comprising 144 square kilometres of South London, divided it into 576 squares of 1/4 square kilometre each, and counted the number of squares containing 0, 1, 2, 3, ... etc., flying bombs.

Total number of hits	537
Number of areas	576
Mean number of hits per area	$\mu = 0.9323$

Table 2.2. Frequency distribution of German V2 bomb-hits in South London

Frequency distribution		Number of areas with N bomb-hits	
N	F_N	Expected [i]	Observed
0	0.394	226.7	229
1	0.367	211.4	211 (211)
2	0.171	98.5	93 (93x2)
3	0.053	30.6	35 (35x3)
4	0.012	7.1	7 (7x4)
5 and over	0.003	1.6	1 (1x7) [ii]
	1	575.9	576 (537)

(i) The reader might wish to refer to this table after becoming acquainted with the procedure for calculating the 'expected' number of hits, as explained in Chapter 3.

(ii) In one area there were seven hits which enter the group '5 and over'.

The table indicates homogeneity over the area and a good conformity to the Poisson law.

2.8   Luria and Delbrück's fluctuation test

Luria and Delbrück (1943) wanted to determine whether the variants of bacteria which were resistant to phage infection were induced as a consequence of interaction with phage, or alternatively, whether they were already present in the culture prior to the addition of phage (acquired resistance hypothesis vs. mutation hypothesis). According to the 'acquired resistance hypothesis' each bacterium in a culture had a certain probability of becoming a resistant variant upon contact with the phage; therefore, over a large number of cultures the number of variants per culture should have been Poisson distributed. According to the 'mutation hypothesis' the variants arose spontaneously during the growth of the culture. In some cultures the mutation would have occurred early and given rise to a very large clone of variants; in others the mutation would have occurred just before selection (addition of the phage) and there would be only one or two resistant variants; and finally in some instances no mutation would have occurred at all. Therefore, the mutation hypothesis predicted that the distribution would be much more 'spread out' than the Poisson; i.e. it would have a *large variance*.

Table 2.3. The number of resistant bacteria in different samples from the same culture

Sample number	Resistant colonies	x_i^2
1	46	2116
2	56	3136
3	52	2704
4	48	2304
5	65	4225
6	44	1936
7	49	2401
8	51	2601
9	56	3136
10	47	2209
mean = 51.4	$\Sigma = 514$	$\Sigma = 26768$

$$V = \frac{\Sigma x_i^2 - \dfrac{(\Sigma x_i)^2}{n}}{n-1} = \frac{26768 - \dfrac{(514)^2}{10}}{9} = 38.7$$

Table 2.4. The number of resistant bacteria in a series of similar cultures

Culture number	Resistant colonies	x_i^2
1	30	900
2	10	100
3	40	1600
4	45	2025
5	183	33489
6	12	144
7	173	29929
8	23	529
9	57	3249
10	51	2601
mean = 62.4	$\Sigma = 624$	$\Sigma = 74566$

$$V = \frac{74566 - \dfrac{(624)^2}{10}}{9} = 3958.7$$

The above experiment was designed to distinguish between the 'acquired resistance hypothesis' and the 'mutation hypothesis'. Once the mutation hypothesis was proven (variance was larger than the mean by several orders of magnitude: 3959 vs. 62) the mutation frequencies could be estimated using the Poisson distribution.

While the number of mutant cells per culture is not Poisson distributed (it is clonally distributed), the number of mutational events (that is, the number of clones of mutants) is Poisson distributed.

In one of their experiments, out of 87 cultures there were 29 cultures where no resistant bacteria were found. The cell input was 2.4×10^8 per culture. The mutation rate was calculated as follows:

$$F_0 = \frac{29}{87} = 0.33$$

$$F_0 = e^{-\mu}$$

$$\mu = -\ln F_0 = -\ln 0.33 = 1.1$$

$$\text{mutation rate} = \frac{1.1 \text{ mutants}}{2.4 \times 10^8 \text{ input}} = 0.46 \times 10^{-8}$$

The reader might want to return to this after reading section 3.6.

2.9   Schrödinger's 'What is Life?'

Schrödinger's green booklet (1944) was highly influential in the forties: it provided the impetus for physicists to start showing an interest in biology (disillusionment with physics because of the atom bomb; Feld and Szillard, 1972) and it inspired a number of non-biologists to enter the new field.

The following quote from Schrödinger's book refers to *variance* and *standard deviation*, although Schrödinger avoids using these two expressions (having in mind the layman readership):

> 'I should like to add one very important quantitative statement concerning the degree of inaccuracy to be expected in any physical law, the so-called √n law. If I tell you that a certain gas under certain conditions of pressure and temperature has a certain density, and if I expressed this by saying that within a certain volume (of a size relevant for some experiment) there are under these conditions just *n* molecules of the gas, then you might be sure that if you could test my statement in a particular moment of time, you would find it inaccurate, the departure being of the order of √n. Hence if the number is *n* = 100, you would find a departure of about 10, thus relative error = 10%. But if *n* = 1 million, you would be likely to find a departure of about 1000, thus relative error = 1/10%. Now, roughly speaking, this statistical law is quite general.'

This mathematical principle is a cornerstone of many of the arguments later developed in this book.

3   Theory

3.1   Distributions

3.1.1   Distributions in general and distributions of cells in particular

If this book were simply about probabilities and statistics, we could have joined forces with those authors who explain distribution theories in the standard manner, giving as examples coin-tossing, dice-throwing or drawing balls from a box. As this book concentrates on biological procedures related to cellular interactions, our examples and results refer to cells.

In order not to limit our examples too much, we should be aware of the fact that phages, cDNAs or other (discretely countable) biological carriers are also well represented by the analyses given in this book. We will be confronted with the word 'distribution' in several different contexts, so let us start by bringing some order into the meaning of the basic definitions. According to *Encyclopedia Britannica* (the favoured 11th edition, 1911) 'distribution' means *spreading out* (from Latin 'distribuere', to deal out). When we assemble and present raw data in experimental research, we are dealing with *numerical distribution*. When we create a framework for theoretical analysis of the numerical distribution we obtain *probability distribution*.

We shall turn our attention to cells in order to explain numerical distribution and probability distribution. After dispensing 10 cells into 10 culture wells, results such as these might be obtained:

Well number	1	2	3	4	5	6	7	8	9	10
Number of cells in a given well	1	0	2	1	0	0	1	1	3	1

This is a numerical distribution.
On counting the fraction of wells:

3/10 of wells contain	0 cells
5/10 of wells contain	1 cell
1/10 of wells contain	2 cells
1/10 of wells contain	3 cells

This is a probability distribution.

3.1.2   *Discrete and continuous distributions*

There are two categories of distribution:

discrete distribution

continuous distribution

Discrete data only take certain values, such as 0, 1, 2, 3 ... etc., or 0.2, 0.4, 0.6, 0.8 ... etc., while continuous data take any value, such as 1.4765, 1.2324 ... etc.

Here are some examples of distributions in each of the two categories:

Discrete distribution	*Continuous distribution*
Number of cells in a sample (N_c)	Amount of protein in a sample (ng)
Number of responding cultures (w_R)	Size of cells (ø μm)
Number of different molecular species of cDNA in a library (N)	Length of time for cell replication (min)

Clearly the amount of protein in a sample is continuously distributed (the diameter of cells is continuously distributed as well, although very small and very large cells might be inconceivable; within a reasonable range any value can be expected). The accuracy of the measuring instruments determines, of course, the precision of the measurements. If we record with great precision, then indeed 'any value' can occur. If we decide 'to lump together' certain values, i.e. use some intervals of measuring (any given range as one group), we obtain a discrete distribution instead of a continuous one.

In practice, continuous variates do not exist, as all measured values are rounded values. In this case the measured value changes at discrete intervals and this variable is called 'granulated'. Granulated variables are actually continuous variables that have been converted into discrete variables by being rounded off. In the case of discrete variables, the same value may occur twice or more. This is almost impossible in the case of continuous variables, but it occurs more often in 'coarsely granulated' measurements. If two or more identical values occur in a sample of a granulated variable they are known as 'ties' or tied values.

All these distinctions between continuous vs. discrete distributions should not take our attention away from the fact that the frequency distribution of cells is a discrete distribution. We will study models which best describe this.

3.1.3   Models of discrete distributions

The distribution of *cells* is a proper example of a *discrete* distribution. We will deal with the discrete distributions of cells here and in most chapters of the book. Before describing the model in detail, we should remind ourselves that the other category of distribution, i.e. continuous distribution, will also have to be scrutinised, as several of the tests which we will learn about and adopt, e.g. tests of significance or the chi-squared test, are based on continuous distributions. In section 4.3 we shall take up the issue of *continuous distributions* again.

An example of a discrete distribution is already given above. When 10 cells were distributed into 10 wells we obtained the following result:

Experiment A:

Well number		1	2	3	4	5	6	7	8	9	10
Number of cells in a given well		1	0	2	1	0	0	1	1	3	1

Without delving too deeply into the area of probabilities, we can accept this result at face value. But how would we judge the following two results?

Experiment B:

Number of cells in a given well	1	1	1	1	1	1	1	1	1	1

Experiment C:

Number of cells in a given well	0	0	0	0	0	0	1	8	1	0

To correctly reflect an actual laboratory result, let us assume again that we have 10 cells in a volume of 100 µl, and dispense 10 µl into each culture well until the suspension is used up. Are experiments B and C plausible? Not at all. Experiment B does not seem like a *random* distribution. In fact, similar results can be obtained with a special type of cell sorter capable of making so-called single cell depositions, i.e. exactly the opposite of random steps. And what about experiment C? This too is not a 'random and independent' distribution. It looks more as if 'clumps' or 'aggregates' rather than single cells were pipetted.

We are intuitively pleased with experiment A, while experiments B and C appear to be improbable. However, we cannot work on the basis of whether we 'intuitively' trust or distrust the outcome. We need to objectively evaluate the results. We shall therefore calculate the theoretical distribution and determine whether or not the experimental outcome can be reconciled with its theoretical counterpart.

The model which describes the distribution of a known number of cells into a fixed number of wells is called the *binomial distribution*. We shall derive the binomial distribution and explain its properties. We will be able to show that experiment A is fully compatible with the rules of the binomial distribution, while experiments B and C represent highly improbable events.

After we have understood the principles of binomial distribution, we will go on to show that yet another type of distribution exists which describes random and independent events: it is called Poisson distribution. We will show that the two distributions are related and we will describe the conditions for which the use of the Poisson distribution is recommended. We will discover that it is simpler to work with the Poisson distribution and more convenient to visualise the graphic representation of the results.

Let us now derive the binomial distribution.

3.2   Binomial distribution

3.2.1   *Product of probabilities*

We will not reiterate our familiar experiment of distributing 10 cells into 10 wells, as we intend to derive a *general formula* for binomial distribution. Thus, we need to know the rules for distributing c cells into w wells. In the word 'binomial', the prefix 'bi-' indicates that each event has two possible outcomes. The cell *succeeds* in falling into a well or *fails* to do so. Therefore we adopt the terms *success* and *failure*. The probability that a cell falls into a given well is high when there are only a few wells to fall into and low when the number of wells is large. The probability p (probability of success) is the reciprocal value of the number of wells, $p = 1/w$. Of course the probability q (probability of failure) is $q = 1 - (1/w)$. The sum of p and q is equal to one, as by definition there is a 100% probability that a cell either falls into a well or does not fall into a well (remembering the prefix 'bi-' there is no other choice).

Having defined c, w, p and q, we need one additional characteristic and this is the effective number of cells in a well. We know that the total number of cells is c, and we define the actual number of cells in a given well to be r. We can find out how many wells remain empty ($r = 0$), or how many contain one ($r = 1$) or two ($r = 2$) cells. The final outcome of the distribution is a product of the probabilities of success p^r and failure q^{c-r}. Therefore the overall probability can be written as

$$p^r \, q^{c-r}$$

However, as we ignored the fact that there are several 'combinatorial' ways to arrive at the given number of successes and failures, one problem still remains. If we say that in a given well there are two cells, it can be cell number one plus cell number two, but it could also be $1 + 3$, or $5 + 9$, etc. This number of different ways is given by the term

$$\frac{c!}{r!(c-r)!}$$

The binomial distribution is defined by the multiplication product of the above two terms

$$P_r = \frac{c!}{r!(c-r)!} \, p^r \, q^{c-r}$$

The combinatorial term is called the binomial coefficient and will be dealt with later when solving a practical problem with the help of Pascal's triangle (see Appendix).

3.2.2 *Parameters* c, w *and* r

Both the binomial and the Poisson distribution are discrete probability distributions. We shall consider three parameters: c, w and r :

c : number of cells to be distributed

w : number of wells into which the cells are distributed

r : number of cells present in a given well

Both c and w are fixed finite integers, r is 0, 1, 2, 3 ... cells. We now distribute c cells into w wells to ascertain what the probability is that a given well contains exactly r cells. The probability that a given cell goes into the chosen well is

$$\frac{1}{w}$$

Therefore the probability that it misses the chosen well is

$$1 - \frac{1}{w}$$

These two values $\frac{1}{w}$ and $1 - \frac{1}{w}$ correspond to 'success' and 'failure' in the probability calculations and are labelled p and q. Thus

$$p = \frac{1}{w}$$

$$q = 1 - \frac{1}{w}$$

$$p + q = 1$$

The standard form of the binomial distribution is

$$P_r = \frac{c!}{r!(c-r)!} p^r q^{c-r}$$

The Poisson distribution also deals with the entities c, w, r, although the fraction $\frac{c}{w}$ is more commonly called μ, which is the average number of cells per well. Then the Poisson distribution is $F_r = \frac{\mu^r}{r!} e^{-\mu}$ and the relationship between these two distributions will become clear in section 3.5.

3.2.3   *Step by step derivation*

We randomly and independently distribute c cells into w wells, and note that the probability that a given cell falls into a chosen well is

$$p = \frac{1}{w} \qquad q = 1 - \frac{1}{w}$$

which are the probabilities of *hit* and *miss* (success and failure). As we know that the probability that a *given* cell falls into a *given* well is $p = \frac{1}{w}$ and that it misses the chosen well is $q = 1 - \frac{1}{w}$, we can establish the probability that all cells miss the chosen well.

What is the probability that all cells miss the chosen well? As the cells are distributed independently and randomly, the probability that they all miss the chosen well is the multiplication product of the probabilities that each one misses

$$P_0 = \left(1 - \frac{1}{w}\right)^c$$

What is the probability that one out of c cells enters, and the others miss the chosen well? The probability that the first cell goes into, and the remainder miss the chosen well is

$$\frac{1}{w}\left(1 - \frac{1}{w}\right)^{c-1}$$

In fact, this is also the probability that the second cell, or the third cell, etc., goes into the chosen well. Thus we must multiply the above term by c

$$P_1 = \frac{c}{w}\left(1 - \frac{1}{w}\right)^{c-1}$$

What is the probability that two cells go into, and $c-2$ cells miss a given well? The term

$$\left(\frac{1}{w}\right)^2 \left(1 - \frac{1}{w}\right)^{c-2}$$

shows the probability that the first cell *and* the second cell go into the chosen well while the remainder miss that given well.

But this is also the probability that the first *and* the third cell, or the second *and* the fourth cell go into the chosen well. Thus we have to multiply the above expression by the number of possible pairs. In this case the number of possible pairs is

$$\frac{c\,(c-1)}{2}$$

Note that c is multiplied by $(c-1)$ because one given cell does not form a pair with 'itself'. Further, the expression is divided by 2, because cell 'one' and cell 'three' is the same pair as cell 'three' and cell 'one'. It follows that

$$P_2 = \frac{c(c-1)}{2}\left(\frac{1}{w}\right)^2\left(1-\frac{1}{w}\right)^{c-2}$$

In the same way we can calculate the probability that three cells go into, and $c-3$ cells miss a given well

$$P_3 = \frac{c(c-1)(c-2)}{3\times 2}\left(\frac{1}{w}\right)^3\left(1-\frac{1}{w}\right)^{c-3}$$

For r cells we can calculate

$$P_r = \frac{c(c-1)(c-2)...(c-r+1)}{r!}\left(\frac{1}{w}\right)^r\left(1-\frac{1}{w}\right)^{c-r}$$

The above equation represents the so-called binomial distribution, although in this form it is hardly recognisable. We proceed to transform it into the 'standard form'. We expand the formula by the quotient

$$\frac{(c-r)(c-r-1)...3\times 2\times 1}{(c-r)(c-r-1)...3\times 2\times 1}$$

and we get

$$P_r = \frac{c(c-1)(c-2)...(c-r+1)}{r!}\frac{(c-r)(c-r-1)...3\times 2\times 1}{(c-r)(c-r-1)...3\times 2\times 1}\left(\frac{1}{w}\right)^r\left(1-\frac{1}{w}\right)^{c-r}$$

and we recognise that the numerator is equal to $c!$, and one part of the denominator is equal to $(c-r)!$ Thus

$$P_r = \frac{c!}{r!(c-r)!}\left(\frac{1}{w}\right)^r\left(1-\frac{1}{w}\right)^{c-r}$$

Throughout the whole derivation we have avoided the well-known 'abstract terms' of p and q as probabilities of 'success' and 'failure', but we have stated at the beginning of the section that

$$\frac{1}{w} \quad \text{and} \quad 1-\frac{1}{w}$$

are probabilities having these properties. It follows that

$$P_r = \frac{c!}{r!(c-r)!}\,p^r\,q^{c-r}$$

which is the standard form of the binomial distribution. For completeness we also give the 'alternative' standard notation

$$P_r = \binom{c}{r} p^r q^{c-r}$$

where $\binom{c}{r} = \dfrac{c!}{r!(c-r)!}$, the so-called binomial coefficient.

3.3   Mean, variance and standard deviation

3.3.1   *Mean*

In the binomial distribution we have taken into consideration the number of cells c and the number of wells w, and have disregarded the relationship between these two parameters, the so-called *mean*. The mean is simply the numerical average of all observations.

For the distribution which we examined earlier, experiment A yielded the following outcome

Well number	1	2	3	4	5	6	7	8	9	10
Number of cells in a given well (r)	1	0	2	1	0	0	1	1	3	1

The population mean is given by $\mu = \Sigma r / w$ (where $\Sigma r = c$)

$$\mu = \frac{1+0+2+1+0+0+1+1+3+1}{10} = 1$$

For the other two examples, B and C, with outcomes

Number of cells in a given well	1	1	1	1	1	1	1	1	1	1

Number of cells in a given well	0	0	0	0	0	0	1	8	1	0

the population mean is

$$\mu = \frac{1+1+1+1+1+1+1+1+1+1}{10} = 1$$

$$\mu = \frac{0+0+0+0+0+0+1+8+1+0}{10} = 1$$

There is another formula for calculating the mean:

$$\mu = 0F_0 + 1F_1 + 2F_2 + 3F_3 + \cdots$$
$$\mu = \Sigma r F_r$$

where $F_0, F_1, F_2, F_3 \cdots$ is the portion of wells containing 0, 1, 2, 3... cells.

In experiment A the calculation is as follows:

3 wells remained empty, i.e. $F_0 = \frac{3}{10} = 0.3$

5 wells received 1 cell, i.e. $F_1 = \frac{5}{10} = 0.5$

1 well received 2 cells, i.e. $F_2 = \frac{1}{10} = 0.1$ and

1 well received 3 cells, i.e. $F_3 = \frac{1}{10} = 0.1$

$$\mu - F_1 + 2F_2 + 3F_3 = 0.5 + 2 \times 0.1 + 3 \times 0.1 = 1$$

For experiments B and C the population mean is

$$\mu = F_1 = 1 \quad \text{(exp. B)}$$
$$\mu = F_1 + 8F_8 = 0.2 + 8 \times 0.1 = 1 \quad \text{(exp. C)}$$

These three outcomes, A, B and C, have a mean equal to *one*, although the distributions are profoundly different. We assume that experiment A fulfils the criteria for random and independent distribution and we suspect that experiments B and C do not, but we need to develop objective criteria for identifying which is which.

3.3.2 *Variance*

Which of the following experiments, A, B and C, displays the largest variation?

	Well number	1	2	3	4	5	6	7	8	9	10
A	Number of cells in a given well	1	0	2	1	0	0	1	1	3	1
B	Number of cells in a given well	1	1	1	1	1	1	1	1	1	1
C	Number of cells in a given well	0	0	0	0	0	0	1	8	1	0

To answer this question we will develop a statistical measure of variation. It will take into account the values of all observations and will express the variation relative to the mean.

The population mean is given by

$$\mu = \frac{\Sigma r}{w} = \frac{c}{w}$$

For A, B and C the population mean is $\mu = \frac{10}{10} = 1$.

In the next step we will try to determine how far each observation lies from the mean. We shall construct a table in which we enter the distance between the observation and the mean. The well with 3 cells will be '2 cells distant' from the average. The largest distance is in the well where 8 cells were found (well number 8 of experiment C); the distance to the mean is *seven*. Empty wells will have a distance of *minus one* (–1).

Table 3.1. The distance between r and μ

Experiment A		Experiment B		Experiment C	
No. of cells in a well	Distance between r and μ	No. of cells in a well	Distance between r and μ	No. of cells in a well	Distance between r and μ
0	$0 - 1 = -1$	1	$1 - 1 = 0$	0	$0 - 1 = -1$
0	$0 - 1 = -1$	1	$1 - 1 = 0$	0	$0 - 1 = -1$
0	$0 - 1 = -1$	1	$1 - 1 = 0$	0	$0 - 1 = -1$
1	$1 - 1 = 0$	1	$1 - 1 = 0$	0	$0 - 1 = -1$
1	$1 - 1 = 0$	1	$1 - 1 = 0$	0	$0 - 1 = -1$
1	$1 - 1 = 0$	1	$1 - 1 = 0$	0	$0 - 1 = -1$
1	$1 - 1 = 0$	1	$1 - 1 = 0$	0	$0 - 1 = -1$
1	$1 - 1 = 0$	1	$1 - 1 = 0$	1	$1 - 1 = 0$
2	$2 - 1 = 1$	1	$1 - 1 = 0$	1	$1 - 1 = 0$
3	$3 - 1 = 2$	1	$1 - 1 = 0$	8	$8 - 1 = 7$
	$\Sigma = 0$		$\Sigma = 0$		$\Sigma = 0$

Note that the sum of the distances is *always* zero. $\Sigma (r - \mu) = 0$. This is true for all three experiments and by definition it is true for all experiments.

In the next step we eliminate the *sign* involved in these differences $(r - \mu)$ by squaring the differences $(r - \mu)^2$. Then we sum up all the squared differences.

Table 3.2. Squared differences

Experiment A			Experiment B			Experiment C		
No. of cells in a well	$r - \mu$	$(r - \mu)^2$	No. of cells in a well	$r - \mu$	$(r - \mu)^2$	No. of cells in a well	$r - \mu$	$(r - \mu)^2$
0	−1	1	1	0	0	0	−1	1
0	−1	1	1	0	0	0	−1	1
0	−1	1	1	0	0	0	−1	1
1	0	0	1	0	0	0	−1	1
1	0	0	1	0	0	0	−1	1
1	0	0	1	0	0	0	−1	1
1	0	0	1	0	0	0	−1	1
1	0	0	1	0	0	1	0	0
2	1	1	1	0	0	1	0	0
3	2	4	1	0	0	8	7	49
		$\Sigma = 8$			$\Sigma = 0$			$\Sigma = 56$

The sum of the squared distances $\Sigma(r-\mu)^2$ is for

Experiment A	8
Experiment B	0
Experiment C	56

And as a final step, we divide this sum by the number of wells. The result which we obtain is the so-called variance

$$V = \frac{\Sigma(r-\mu)^2}{w}$$

Experiment A	$V = 0.8$
Experiment B	$V = 0$
Experiment C	$V = 5.6$

The value of the variance V is highly informative, it tells us whether or not the elements of the distribution were assorted randomly and independently, or not. We shall see in later chapters that for the types of distribution which obey the Poisson law the variance is numerically equal to the mean. From the above three experiments it is the variance in experiment A ($V = 0.8$) which is quite similar to the mean ($\mu = 1$).

3.3.3 Standard deviation

Variance is a very good measure of the variation in the analysed (cell) population. Necessarily we have to introduce yet another definition, the *standard deviation* (σ). The standard deviation is defined as the square root of variance

$$V = \frac{\Sigma(r-\mu)^2}{w}$$

$$\sigma = \sqrt{V} = \sqrt{\frac{\Sigma(r-\mu)^2}{w}}$$

Because of the above relationship between σ and V, variance is often written as sigma square ($V = \sigma^2$).

To reiterate, the variance is the best 'quality control' for the set of observations, since within the framework of random discrete distributions presented in this book the *variance is numerically equal to the mean*.

However, one formal reason exists why we must introduce the term standard deviation, and that is because it is expressed in the same units of measurement as are the observations, and the mean, themselves. Variance and mean cannot be plotted on the same coordinate axis, in the same way that cm^2 and cm cannot be plotted on the same scale.

Advanced

Other aspects of σ, such as Chebyshev's theorem (at least 75% of the observations are found in the range of $\mu - 2\sigma$ and $\mu + 2\sigma$) are beyond the scope of this book.

We recapitulate the equations

mean $\qquad\qquad\qquad\qquad \mu = \dfrac{\Sigma r}{w} = \dfrac{c}{w}$

and also $\qquad\qquad\qquad\quad \mu = F_1 + 2F_2 + 3F_3 + \ldots = \Sigma r F_r$

sum of the distances of
observations to the mean $\qquad \Sigma (r - \mu) = 0$

variance $\qquad\qquad\qquad\quad V = \dfrac{\Sigma (r - \mu)^2}{w}$

standard deviation $\qquad\quad\ \sigma = \sqrt{V}$

where w is the number of wells, and r is the actual number of cells in a given well.

For experiments A, B and C we obtain

Table 3.3. Variance and standard deviation

	Experiment A	Experiment B	Experiment C
Number of cells (c)	10	10	10
Number of wells (w)	10	10	10
Mean (μ)	1	1	1
Sum of the distances $\Sigma (r - \mu)$	0	0	0
Variance (V)	0.8	0	5.6
Standard deviation (σ)	0.89	0	2.37

3.4   The constant e and its reciprocal value

3.4.1   *The constant* e

Throughout this book we will be using a constant called e, the value of which is about 2.7. Besides the constant e, we will also use the reciprocal value of the number e:

$$e = 2.71828$$

$$\frac{1}{e} = 0.37\ldots$$

Without having the constant e we could not proceed further, in the same way that geometry problems cannot be approached without the constant π.

The constant e also serves as a base for the so-called *natural logarithm*, whereby

$$\ln_e e = 1$$

3.4.2 Maclaurin series

Maclaurin worked with the infinite series

$$\frac{\mu^0}{0!}, \frac{\mu^1}{1!}, \frac{\mu^2}{2!}, \frac{\mu^3}{3!}, \frac{\mu^4}{4!}, \cdots$$

He showed that for the special case of $\mu = 1$, the sum of the series equals a constant which can be calculated as precisely as required.

The general form of the sum of the Maclaurin series is

$$e^\mu = \frac{\mu^0}{0!} + \frac{\mu^1}{1!} + \frac{\mu^2}{2!} + \frac{\mu^3}{3!} + \frac{\mu^4}{4!} + \cdots$$

and for $\mu = 1$

$$e = 1 + 1 + \frac{1}{2!} + \frac{1}{3!} + \frac{1}{4!} + \cdots \approx 2.71828$$

3.4.3 Reciprocal value of e

In the branch of calculus dealing with *limits*, expressions such as

$$\lim_{x \to \infty} \left(1 - \frac{1}{x}\right) = 1$$

are often used. The meaning of the above term is that if in the fraction $1 - \frac{1}{x}$, a very large x is used, the value of the term will be close to *one*.

Standard procedures exist for deriving the limits. Calculus books include lists of limit solutions. One example is shown below. It differs from the previous one in that the fraction $1 - \frac{1}{x}$ is raised to the power of x.

$$\lim_{x \to \infty} \left(1 - \frac{1}{x}\right)^x = e^{-1}$$

We have already worked with a similar expression

$$\left(1 - \frac{1}{w}\right)^c$$

in which c was the number of cells and w the number of wells. For a special situation, when the number of cells c and the number of wells w is equal (thus when the mean number of cells per well is *one*, $\mu = \frac{c}{w} = 1$) we are entitled to say

$$\left(1-\frac{1}{w}\right)^{c}=\left(1-\frac{1}{w}\right)^{w}=\left(1-\frac{1}{c}\right)^{c}$$

then the

$$\lim_{w\to\infty}\left(1-\frac{1}{w}\right)^{w}=\lim_{c\to\infty}\left(1-\frac{1}{c}\right)^{c}=e^{-1}=\frac{1}{e}$$

If the reader has some spare time and a calculator on hand, he/she might want to calculate the following terms

$$\left(\tfrac{3}{4}\right)^{4},\quad\left(\tfrac{4}{5}\right)^{5}\dots,\quad\left(\tfrac{9}{10}\right)^{10},\quad\left(\tfrac{19}{20}\right)^{20},\quad\left(\tfrac{99}{100}\right)^{100}$$

The results asymptotically approach the above-mentioned value of

$$\tfrac{1}{e}\approx 0.369$$

The general form of the limit is

$$\lim_{w\to\infty}\left(1-\frac{1}{w}\right)^{c}=e^{-\frac{c}{w}}$$

3.5   Poisson distribution

3.5.1   *From binomial to Poisson*

We shall soon see that it is convenient to leave the binomial distribution behind and switch to a similar – but in many respects simpler – model called Poisson distribution. The fundamental assumptions underlying both distributions are very similar.

In both models c cells are randomly and independently distributed into w wells, though in the Poisson model we 'lump' the c and the w into the *mean number of cells per well*, termed $\mu=\tfrac{c}{w}$.

Both the *binomial* and the *Poisson* distribution allow the number of wells to be calculated which contain no cells, or 1, 2, 3, 4 ... cells, but the calculation via the *Poisson* model is much simpler. The graphic representation of the data is also much simpler.

3.5.2   *Derivation of the zero term*

The binomial distribution $P_{r}=\dfrac{c!}{r!(c-r)!}\,p^{r}\,q^{c-r}$

where P_{r} is the probability that r cells are present in a given well *r* is the number of cells (in a given well)

c is the number of cells

$$p = \frac{1}{w}, \quad q = 1 - \frac{1}{w}, \text{ where } w \text{ is the number of wells}$$

The fraction of wells in which no cells can be found is

$$P_0 = \frac{c!}{0!\,(c-0)!} \, p^0 \, q^{t-0}$$

$$P_0 = \quad 1 \quad \times 1 \times q^c$$

$$P_0 = \left(1 - \frac{1}{w}\right)^c$$

We have seen in the section 3.4.3 that

$$\lim_{w \to \infty} \left(1 - \frac{1}{w}\right)^c = e^{-\frac{c}{w}}$$

One of the features of the transition from the binomial to the Poissonian model is the use of the *mean number of cells per well* (μ) instead of the number of cells (c) and the number of wells (w).

$$\mu = \frac{c}{w}$$

Thus we have derived the zero term of the Poisson distribution

$$F_0 = e^{-\mu}$$

We decided to use P_0 (P for probability) in the binomial model, while reserving F_0 (F for fraction) for use in the Poissonian model. Obviously, when the two models converge, the probability P_0 and the fraction F_0 also converge ($P_0 = F_0$).

3.5.3 Step by step derivation

For all practical purposes we know that both the number of cells c and the number of wells w are large, but conceptually we can consider them still many-fold larger. In other words, although we use a pool of mouse spleens for the preparation of a cell suspension, we can imagine that this itself is a 'homogeneous' sample from all available mice, and the few hundred culture wells which are filled with these cells are themselves a fair representation of the many thousands of wells which could have been set up.

In any case it is clear that it is not the absolute number of cells distributed which is important but the ratio of cells per well. The ratio of the number c cells distributed into w wells is the mean μ

Advanced

However, in most applications in experimental science, our task will be to estimate the μ from an experimentally detected *zero* term of the Poisson distribution. This will be shown below in section 3.7.2. Special circumstances exist in which the higher terms (e.g. the second and third terms) are known. In section 3.7.3 the procedure will be shown for calculating μ from these terms.

We could ask why, in this book, should we develop the argument of using various cell dilutions if the frequency can be directly estimated from a single data set. The answer is that the direct calculation is only valid if the experimental system 'obeys the rules' of so-called single-hit kinetics. Although there will be a full explanation on hits and targets, a brief guiding rule may be mentioned now. Direct calculation of μ from a single data set (i.e. from a single dilution, for example, from the number of nonresponding cultures obtained in sixty cultures) is permitted if we can assume that only the analysed cell type (the titrated cell type, e.g. B cells) is limiting and all other components (T cells, antigen-presenting cells) are in excess. Data from a single cell concentration *never* show whether these conditions are fulfilled, while a titration in which several cell dilutions are used *always* shows when deviation from single-hit kinetics occurs (see Chapters 5 and 6).

3.7.2   Calculation of μ from known F_0

The zero term of the Poisson distribution is

$$F_0 = e^{-\mu}$$

We modify the equation in such a manner that we 'logarithm' both sides of the equations

$$\ln F_0 = \ln e^{-\mu}$$

which can be written as

$$\ln F_0 = -\mu \times \ln e$$

Since $\ln e$ is equal to one we are entitled to write

$$\mu = -\ln F_0$$

Using a pocket calculator, we enter the value F_0, find the natural logarithm, and the negative value of the result is the μ estimate.

For example, we have set up 60 cultures at a cell density of 30 000 cells/well, and upon stimulation with antigen we obtained 10 responding cultures

$$F_0 = \frac{50}{60} = 0.83$$

$$\mu = -\ln F_0 = -\ln 0.83 = 0.16$$

Thus, 30 000 cells contain on average 0.16 precursor cells. The frequency is

$$f = \frac{0.16}{30\,000} = 5.2 \times 10^{-6}$$

We can phrase it as follows: there are 5.2 precursor cells per million cells. Another form of the (same) statement is: there is 1 precursor cell per 190 000 cells.

3.7.3 Calculation of μ from higher terms

There are special circumstances in which the value of F_0 is not known, while higher terms of the Poisson distribution are known. Before giving an example we shall show the calculation.

The first and the second terms of the Poisson distribution are:

$$F_1 = \mu \, e^{-\mu}$$

$$F_2 = \frac{\mu^2}{2} e^{-\mu}$$

We divide the two terms:

$$\frac{F_2}{F_1} = \frac{\dfrac{\mu^2}{2} e^{-\mu}}{\mu \, e^{-\mu}} = \frac{\mu}{2}$$

$$\text{and } \mu = 2F_2/F_1$$

Example

It is generally assumed that in a living cell, the members of a mRNA population are not present at equal frequencies. If the diverse populations of mRNA were present at equal frequencies, we could then calculate the number of expected occurrences in 'partitioned' collections of cDNA clones (pools). In our readout system (2D gels of the cell-free expression products of individual pools) we record the presence of the gene products. Since our data do not contain the zero term of the Poisson distribution, we can establish the mean number of cDNA clones (here cDNA or mRNA can be used in the same argument) from $F_1 = \mu \, e^{-\mu}$ and $F_2 = \left(\mu^2 / 2!\right) e^{-\mu}$. The fractions F_1 and F_2 signify the proportion of clones present on one and two gels, respectively, and μ is the mean number of clones in a pool.

Data: 816 singles (i.e. present on any of the gels once)
                412 doubles (i.e. present on any two combinations of gels)

$$\mu = 2\frac{F_2}{F_1} = 2\frac{412}{846} = 0.974$$

The calculated value of μ ($\mu = 0.974$) describes a distribution ($F_0 = 0.38$, $F_1 = 0.37$, $F_2 = 0.18$, $F_3 = 0.06$) which can be compared to the experimental findings (Lefkovits *et al.*, 1995).

Advanced

3.8   Graphical representation of the Poisson distribution

3.8.1   *The semi-log plot*

We have explained how one can estimate the parameter μ from a known value of F_0, and we have warned that such a calculation is only correct when certain conditions are fulfilled. We will get used to the idea that the experiments have to be planned and executed in such a manner that several different sample inputs are employed for the analyses. This will be explained in detail in other chapters, here we describe the basic features of the resulting plot.

Earlier we learned how to modify the zero term of the Poisson distribution into its logarithmic form, and have written $\mu = -\ln F_0$. In plain language the formula means that the negative logarithm of the fraction of nonresponding cultures is linearly proportional to the mean number of precursor cells per culture. It follows that if we plot the negative logarithm of the fraction of nonresponding cultures ($-\ln F_0$) on the y axis, and the cell input (μ) at the linear scale on the x axis, we expect that the experimental points will fit a straight line passing through the origin.

3.8.2   *37% intercept*

By introducing the semi-log plot we evolve beyond the procedure of estimation of μ from a single value of F_0 and enter the world of limiting dilution (the x axis accommodates several cell inputs).

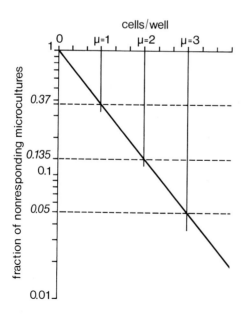

Figure 3.1. Intercepts of the Poisson straight line for $\mu = 1$, $\mu = 2$, $\mu = 3$

Here we show that the semi-log plot offers an 'easy to use' feature for the estimation of μ by interpolation at the 37% intercept. In the zero term of the Poisson distribution $F_0 = e^{-\mu}$, we substitute for $\mu = 1$, and obtain

$$F_0 = e^{-1} = 1/e \approx 0.37$$

The semi-log plot indicates that the intercept of the Poisson straight line with the 37% horizontal line defines the position of $\mu = 1$.

In the figure two other intercepts are indicated

$$\text{for } \mu = 2 \quad F_0 = e^{-\mu} = e^{-2} = 1/e^2 \approx 0.135$$

$$\text{for } \mu = 3 \quad F_0 = e^{-\mu} = e^{-3} = 1/e^3 \approx 0.05$$

The value 0.05 for the mean of *three* is of mnemonic interest and will be dealt with later in the book.

3.8.3 Slope

Estimates of frequencies in a Poissonian analysis can be obtained directly from the graphical representation. The nature of the semi-log plot is such that a steep straight line stands for high frequencies, and a shallow line for low frequencies.

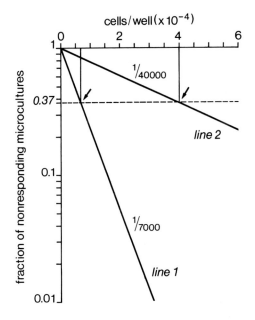

Figure 3.2. Steep and shallow slope of the Poisson straight line

On Figure 3.2 the 37% intercept marks 7000 cells (line 1) and 40 000 cells (line 2)

$$\text{for line 1} \quad f = 1/7000 = 1.42 \times 10^{-4}$$
$$\text{for line 2} \quad f = 1/40\,000 = 2.5 \times 10^{-5}$$

Line 1 stands for a 5.7 times higher frequency than line 2 ($1.42 \times 10^{-4}/2.5 \times 10^{-5}$). It should be noted that the frequency estimate does not need to be read at the intercept: it can be obtained at any portion of the line, because what matters is the slope. Thus, as indicated in Figure 3.3a, instead of 0.37/7000 it can be read at Δ 0.37/Δ 7000. This is of special importance in cases where the experimental points form a straight line which does not pass through the origin, e.g. in measurements with high background detection. In such instances the intercept at 37% does not yield a correct frequency (intercept at 18 000), while the slope is the same for (i) and (ii) (Figure 3.3b).

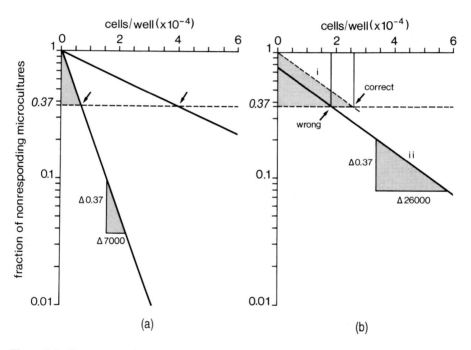

Figure 3.3. Frequency estimate at Δ 0.37. (a) from a straight line through the origin, (b) from a straight line based on measurements with high background detection

4 Statistics

The previous chapter on *distributions* belongs to a branch of mathematics in which statements are *a priori* true. This chapter on *statistics* deals with statements for which one must accept some convenient *ad hoc* principles. Probability and statistics both deal with sampling. In the former, the sampling is theoretical, in the latter, it is empirical. We will describe various tests and procedures with the aim of analysing whether the data fit a certain model, and we will use a judgement of credibility towards the results obtained.

In sections 4.1 and 4.2 we will explain how a straight line is fitted to limiting dilution data on a semi-log plot. Then we describe the use of the chi-squared test of goodness of fit, a type of quality control for the regression lines. Following this we outline a correlation test for comparing several sets of data, and describe Fisher's exact test for independence using 2x2 contingency tables. Furthermore, we will cover the methodology for calculating the confidence limits of the experimental points and the procedure for calculating the confidence limits of the slope.

Two additional procedures for analysing limiting dilution data are given. One is a technique developed by Taswell (1981, 1987) based on minimum chi-squared statistics, while another, originally described by Finney (1951) and adapted by Fazekas (1982), is a maximum likelihood test.

4.1   Linear regression through the origin

From the zero term of the Poisson distribution we can anticipate that the experimental results of a limiting dilution analysis, expressed as the negative logarithm of the fraction of nonresponding cultures, will be linearly proportional to the cell input. In an ideal case, the results will lie on a straight line passing through the origin. We refer to single-hit Poissonian processes, as explained in Chapter 3 (Theory).

Before describing the actual procedure for expressing this linear relationship we provide the following definitions which apply to both this and the next section:

(i)   If we assume that parameters x and y are related in a linear fashion, then the equation

$$y = ax + b$$

describes this relationship.

(ii) In the equation $y = ax + b$

a represents the slope of the line, and

b is the point of the intercept between the line and the y axis (y intercept)

(iii) If we know the values a and b (and we will), we can plug in an arbitrary value for x and determine the value for y. Therefore, the equation for this relationship is called the 'prediction equation'.

(iv) The line defined by the prediction equation is also known as a regression line. It has the property that it passes near the experimental points in the way that best defines the studied process. The regression line need not pass through any of the points to give the best fit for the points plotted.

(v)   To produce the equation we require that the line passes as closely as possible to all points. This can be achieved by making the sum of the distances (experimental points to the line) as small as possible. A more meaningful approach is to minimise the sum of the squares (since the numerical values of the squares are always positive this proposition eliminates the problem that the distances 'above' the regression line are positive, while those 'below' the line are negative [also see sections 3.3.2, 3.3.3 and 3.6.3 on sample variance]).

We will now derive the prediction equation. Let us assume that we obtain a set of data by LDA which can be best described by a straight line through the origin. We assume (or we know) that zero cell input yields no background positive cultures.

Single-hit Poissonian processes in limiting dilution analysis: if we plot the negative logarithm of the fraction of non-responding cultures ($-\ln F_0$) on the y axis, and the cell input (on the linear scale) on the x axis, we expect the experimental points to fit a straight line passing through the origin.

Table 4.1. Results of a B-cell titration

x	y_i		
($\times 10^{-4}$ cells/well)	w_R	F_0	$\ln F_0$
1	18	0.700	− 0.357
2	23	0.617	− 0.483
3	35	0.417	− 0875
4	46	0.233	− 1.455
5	45	0.250	− 1.386
6	55	0.083	− 2.485

$$F_0 = (w_T - w_R) / w_T$$
$$w_T = 60$$

The above data plotted on a semi-log scale are as follows:

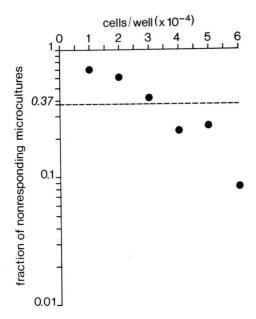

Figure 4.1. Experimental data of a B cell titration displayed on a semi-log scale

We shall now find an estimate $\hat{y}_i$ for each y_i value so that the sum of squares $\Sigma(y_i - \hat{y}_i)^2$ is minimal. The problem can be reduced to finding coefficient a for the function $y = ax$. It can be derived that

$$a = \frac{\Sigma x_i y_i}{\Sigma x_i^2}$$

The set of data in Table 4.1 can be rearranged thus:

Table 4.2. Data for calculating the regression line through the origin

x_i	y_i	$x_i y_i$	x_i^2
1	− 0.357	− 0.357	1
2	− 0.483	− 0.967	4
3	− 0.875	− 2.626	9
4	− 1.455	− 5.821	16
5	− 1.386	− 6.932	25
6	− 2.485	− 14.909	36
		− 31.612	91

$$a = \frac{\Sigma x_i y_i}{\Sigma x_i^2} = \frac{-31.612}{91} = -0.347$$

The straight line through the origin, for which y has the property that the sum of the squares $\Sigma(y_i - \hat{y}_i)^2$ is minimal, is a linear function:

$$y = -0.347\, x$$

The slope –0.347 allows us to construct the straight line. Since the value –0.347 represents $\ln F_0$, it has to be converted to F_0 (it is 0.707) (on a pocket calculator it is keyed in as follows: 0.347, change sign, INV, ln).

4.1.1 *The value of the slope* a *is the frequency*

In the equation $y = ax$, the cell dose x at $y = -1$ (i.e. under the conditions of 37% nonresponding cultures) is a dose containing *one* precursor cell on average. The reciprocal value thereof $(1/x)$ is the frequency

$$y = ax$$
$$-1 = ax$$
$$x = -\frac{1}{a}$$
$$f = \frac{1}{x} = -a$$

(the 'order of magnitude component' has to be included as indicated below). In the prediction equation $y = -0.347\, x$ we will substitute for $y = -1$ (see scale [a] of Figure 4.2) and we obtain $x = \frac{-1}{-0.347}$. To obtain numerically correct frequency values it suffices to include the order of magnitude component, as given in the graphical representation (e.g. 10^{-4}).

Frequency estimate (x 10^4) = 0.347

Frequency estimate f = 0.347 x 10^{-4}

$= 3.47$ x 10^{-5}

$$\frac{1}{f} = \frac{1}{3.47 \times 10^{-5}} = 28\ 800 \text{ cells}$$

cell dose containing 1 precursor cell on average

Calculation of the frequency from the slope of the prediction equation gives the same results as reading from the 37% intercept.

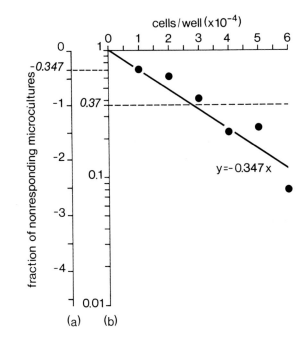

Figure 4.2. Fitting straight line through the origin (in section 4.3 it will be referred to as plot 1). The straight line was fitted by the method of least squares; linear function $y = -0.347\ x$ was converted for plotting into a logarithmic one. a) Logarithmic values on a linear scale. b) Linear values on a logarithmic scale

4.2   Linear regression disregarding the origin

A straight line through the origin is expected when single-hit Poissonian events are recorded (section 5.4). However, there are instances when we have good reason to expect that the data could be explained by a straight line not going through the origin (high background of the measured response, a multi-target event [section 5.6]). In these cases we perform linear regression *disregarding the origin*.

We should be aware of the implications of deriving a prediction equation for a straight line not going through the origin. We do so only if the data cannot be explained by the single-hit Poissonian model. Whether such conditions are met is in most instances clear from the raw data plots, but an objective evaluation is possible by applying tests described later in this chapter (sections 4.3 and 4.7). Here we simply learn the procedure for deriving the prediction equation for a regression line without constraints of the origin.

We will use the same set of data as in section 4.1 (i.e. as in Table 4.1) though here we shall also include Σx_i and Σy_i (which were not needed up to now; compare Table 4.2).

Table 4.3. Data for calculating the regression line disregarding the origin

	x_i	y_i	$x_i y_i$	x_i^2
	1	− 0.357	− 0.357	1
	2	− 0.483	− 0.967	4
	3	− 0.876	− 2.626	9
	4	− 1.455	− 5.821	16
	5	− 1.386	− 6.932	25
$n = 6$	6	− 2.485	− 14.909	36
	21	− 7.042	− 31.612	91

Again, as in section 4.1, we will find an estimate $\hat{y}_i$ for each y_i value so that the sum of squares $\Sigma(y_i - \hat{y}_i)^2$ is minimal. We will consider the linear function

$$y = ax + b$$

in which a is the slope and b is the intercept with the y axis. Values a and b will be calculated from the following two formulae

$$a = \frac{n\Sigma x_i y_i - (\Sigma x_i)(\Sigma y_i)}{n\Sigma x_i^2 - (\Sigma x_i)^2}$$

$$b = \bar{y} - a\bar{x} = \left(\frac{\Sigma y_i}{n}\right) - a\left(\frac{\Sigma x_i}{n}\right)$$

$$a = -\frac{6 \times 31.612 - 21 \times 7.042}{6 \times 91 - 21 \times 21} = -\frac{41.789}{105} = -0.398$$

$$b = -\frac{7.042}{6} + 0.398\frac{21}{6} = -1.174 + 1.393 = 0.219$$

The straight line disregarding the origin, for which y has the property that the sum of the squares $\Sigma(y_i - \hat{y}_i)^2$ is minimal, is a linear function:

$$y = -0.398\ x + 0.219$$

The frequency is calculated from the slope a by the same procedure as described for the prediction equation through the origin; the contribution of b is disregarded. The value at the 37% intercept should not be used for the frequency calculation (the calculation from Δ37% is permitted, as explained in detail in section 3.8.3).

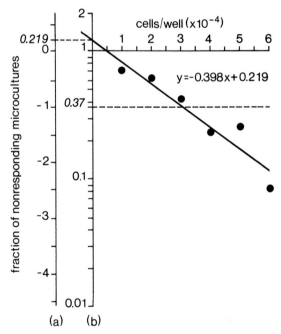

Figure 4.3. Fitting a straight line without the constraints of the origin (in section 4.3 it will be referred to as plot 2). a) Logarithmic values on a linear scale. b) Linear values on a logarithmic scale

For the frequency calculation we formally transpose the line by the value b, so that we consider $y = -0.398x$. Now the arguments are the same as in section 4.1. Here, too, we include the order of the magnitude component as given in the graphical representation (i.e. 10^{-4}).

Frequency estimate (x 10^4)   = 0.398

Frequency estimate $f = 0.398 \times 10^{-4}$

$= 3.98 \times 10^{-5}$

$$\frac{1}{f} = \frac{1}{3.98 \times 10^{-5}} = 25\,100 \text{ cells}$$

cell dose containing 1 precursor cell on average

Note that the 37% intercept reads 30 700, which is incorrect. Reading at Δ 37% (see section 3.8) correctly yields Δ 25 000 cells.

4.3   Chi-squared test for goodness of fit

First we shall explain some basic concepts and provide a few definitions. We already know (section 3.1.2) that there are two categories of distributions: *discrete* and *continuous*. Most of the theoretical background for the limiting dilution analysis – which we have dealt with exhaustively – is based on two types of *discrete distribution*: binomial and Poisson. It turns out that for the analysis of the errors of measurement (mean, variance, standard deviation, confidence limits, etc.) several types of continuous distributions are of importance:

(i)   *normal distribution* is a family of symmetric continuous distributions with two parameters:
  - the mean μ, and
  - the variance σ^2

normal distributions are symmetrical about the mean μ; *standard normal distributions* are symmetrical about $\mu = 0$ and $\sigma^2 = 1$.

(ii) *t-distribution*[*] is a family of symmetric continuous distributions with a single parameter:
  - *df*, which is a positive integer known as the number of degrees of freedom of the distribution. As the *df* increases, the *t*-distribution comes to resemble the standard normal distribution. For the regression line $y = ax$, the *df* equals $n - 1$, while for $y = ax + b$, the *df* equals $n - 2$, where n is the sample size.

t-distributions are symmetrical about 0.

(iii) *chi-squared distribution* is a family of non-symmetrical (skewed) continuous distributions with a single parameter:
  - *df*, which is a positive integer known as the number of degrees of freedom of the distribution. In the chi-squared distributions

---

[*] Developed by Gosset, under the pseudonym 'Student', therefore also known as 'Student's *t*-distribution' (see sections 2.4 and 4.7, and the Appendix).

the amount of *variation* present in the set of observations, rather than the *mean* of the set of observations, is compared.

We will now consider the actual test. In the previous sections we obtained:

- a straight line through the origin, and
- a straight line without constraints of the origin

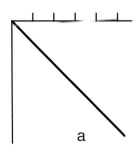
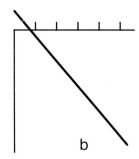

a   b

Figure 4.4. Graphical representation of the prediction equations for linear regression lines through the origin (a), and lines without the constraints of the origin (b). Test for goodness of fit is meant to establish whether or not the regression lines fit the data

The number of responding or nonresponding wells expected from the prediction equations can be calculated (and will be needed later).

Table 4.4. Tabulated values calculated from the prediction equations

	$y = -0.347\,x$				$y = -0.398\,x + 0.219$		
x	$\hat{y}$	$\hat{F}_0$	$\hat{w}_- = 60 \times \hat{F}_0$	x	$\hat{y}$	$\hat{F}_0$	$\hat{w}_- = 60 \times \hat{F}_0$
1	− 0.347	0.707	42.39	1	− 0.179	0.837	50.18
2	− 0.694	0.500	29.95	2	− 0.577	0.562	33.71
3	− 1.042	0.353	21.16	3	− 0.975	0.377	22.64
4	− 1.390	0.250	14.95	4	− 1.373	0.253	15.21
5	− 1.737	0.176	10.56	5	− 1.771	0.170	10.21
6	− 2.084	0.125	7.46	6	− 2.169	0.114	6.86

$\hat{F}_0$ is the fraction of nonresponding cultures based on the $\hat{y}$ values of the prediction equation. $\hat{F}_0$ values can also be read directly from Figures 4.2 and 4.3. Although the straight lines fulfil the requirement that the squares of the distances are minimal, we do not yet know whether or not the fit is good, i.e. whether the model $y = ax$ or $y = ax + b$ is appropriate.

Below we describe a powerful test which enables us to make a judgement on the quality of fit. The test is based on some unique properties of the chi-squared distribution. We shall start with a definition. If random samples of size

n are drawn from a *normal* population with mean μ and variance σ^2, then the quantity

$$\chi^2 = \frac{df \times V}{\sigma^2}$$

is the value of a random variable having a chi-squared distribution with $n - 1$ degrees of freedom. This formula – though developed for the normal distribution – also holds true for variables which are binomially distributed, as is the case in the examples described here. Note that $\sigma^2 = w_T \times p \times q$ and $V =$ observed variance (definitions of observed and true variance [V, σ^2] are given in the box below).

Chi-squared distribution, as can be seen in Figure 4.5, is skewed to the right.

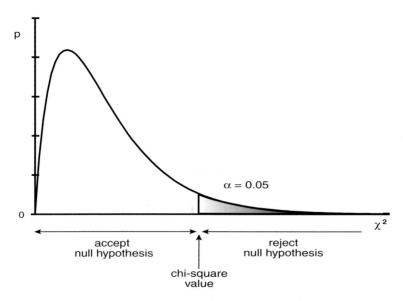

Figure 4.5. Schematic representation of the chi-squared distribution. The null hypothesis states that the data fit the prediction equation. The null hypothesis is rejected if the chi-squared value is larger than the value which defines the tail area of $\alpha = 0.05$. More details are given in the Appendix.

It is customary to use Greek letters for true (but unknown) values, and Latin letters for their estimates (observed values). Thus, variance as a parameter of the normal distribution is called sigma square (σ^2).

true variance = σ^2 while the value which is calculated (observed) is the

estimated variance = V (in many textbooks s^2)

In the equation $\chi^2 = \frac{df \times V}{\sigma^2}$ we recognise that there are two variances, V (observed)

and σ^2 (true).

The calculated χ_i^2 value represents a point on the horizontal axis that defines an area on the long end tail. This area represents a probability p to find by chance a χ^2 value as large as or larger than the observed one. It is customary to conclude that when p is smaller than 0.05, the data deviate in a statistically significant manner from the model (in this case from the prediction equation $y = ax$). In most instances the relationship between the chi-squared values and probabilities are available in computer programs (it is also the case in the LDA program of this monograph). Note that one might want to choose a more significant level e.g. 0.001 (such a choice should be made prior to the evaluation).

An easy-to-use chart of χ^2 values plotted against the probability range from $p = 0.001$ to 1 was published by Bliss in 1944. The chart was reproduced in the first edition of the LDA monograph, and a 'new' version of the chart – recalculated and plotted by Rubes (co-author of the LDA software) is given in the Appendix. A portion of the chart with highlighted curves for 4 and 5 degrees of freedom (as required in the test example) is shown below (Figure 4.6).

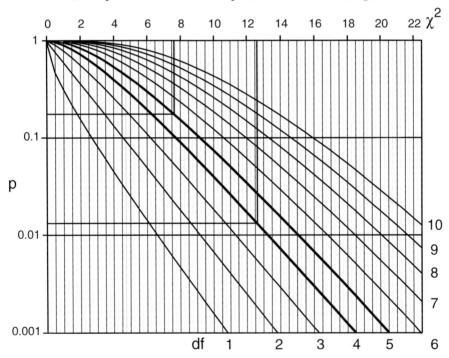

Figure 4.6. A chart showing a portion of chi-squared distribution (see Appendix for full chart). χ^2 distribution is plotted on a semi-logarithmic scale covering a probability range from $p = 0.001$ to 1.0. A separate curve is drawn for each of the degrees of freedom, df 1 to 10. The curves with 4 and 5 degrees of freedom are highlighted. Intercept lines for reading the p values for the two worked examples of Tables 4.5 and 4.6 are indicated.

For the processes depicted on plots 1 and 2 in Figures 4.2 and 4.3 (also schematically represented on Figure 4.4), we formulate the null hypothesis:

Plot 1:   the experimental data conform to single-hit kinetics (model $y = ax$)

Plot 2:   the experimental data conform to the regression line not forced through the origin (model $y = ax + b$)

We shall compose a table in which we enter the following observed and calculated values.

(i)   observed number of responding and nonresponding wells (w_R and w_-)

(ii)   calculated number of responding and nonresponding wells ($\hat{w}_R$ and $\hat{w}_-$) (calculation performed from the prediction equation:
$y = -0.347\,x$, in the case of plot 1, or
$y = -0.398\,x + 0.219$, in the case of plot 2)

(iii)   the difference between observed and calculated values (Δw) is computed (a positive or a negative sign can be entered or disregarded; it is of no consequence since the square of that value is used later)

(iv)   the square of the difference is calculated

(v)   the values $\Delta^2 / \hat{w}_R$ and $\Delta^2 / \hat{w}_-$ are established

(vi)   the sum of these values is χ^2

(vii)   the number of degrees of freedom is established

(for the prediction equation

$y = -0.347\,x$ the number of degrees of freedom is $n - 1$, while for

$y = -0.398\,x + 0.219$ the number of degrees of freedom is $n - 2$).

(viii)   the p value is read from the Bliss/Rubes chart

(ix)   the null hypothesis is or is not rejected

Table 4.5. Display of tabulated data for plot 1

x_i	$y_{i(obs)}$		$\hat{y}_{i(calc)}$		Δw	Δ^2	$\dfrac{\Delta^2}{\hat{w}_R}$	$\dfrac{\Delta^2}{\hat{w}_-}$
	w_R	w_-	$\hat{w}_R$	$\hat{w}_-$				
1	18	42	17.61	42.39	0.39	0.16	0.01	0.00
2	23	37	30.05	29.95	7.05	49.68	1.65	1.66
3	35	25	38.84	21.16	3.84	14.73	0.38	0.70
4	46	14	45.05	14.95	0.95	0.91	0.02	0.06
5	45	15	49.44	10.56	4.44	19.68	0.40	1.86
6	55	5	52.54	7.46	2.46	6.07	0.12	0.81
							2.58	5.09

w_R = responding wells

w_- = nonresponding wells

$\chi^2 = 2.58 + 5.09 = 7.67$

$df = n - 1 = 5$ $\left.\begin{array}{l}\end{array}\right\}$ read the p value from the chart shown on Figure 4.6

$p = 0.19$

Conclusion for plot 1: the null hypothesis is accepted and we consider that the experimental data conform to single-hit kinetics.

Table 4.6. Display of tabulated data for plot 2

x_i	$y_{i(obs)}$		$\hat{y}_{i(calc)}$		Δw	Δ^2	$\dfrac{\Delta^2}{\hat{w}_R}$	$\dfrac{\Delta^2}{\hat{w}_-}$
	w_R	w_-	$\hat{w}_R$	$\hat{w}_-$				
1	18	42	9.82	50.18	8.18	66.93	6.82	1.33
2	23	37	26.29	33.71	3.29	10.86	0.41	0.32
3	35	25	37.36	22.64	2.36	5.58	0.15	0.25
4	46	14	44.79	15.21	1.21	1.45	0.03	0.10
5	45	15	49.79	10.21	4.79	22.91	0.46	2.24
$n = 6$ 6	55	5	53.14	6.86	1.86	3.46	0.07	0.50
							7.94	4.74

$\chi^2 = 7.94 + 4.74 = 12.68$

$df = n - 2 = 4$ $\left.\begin{array}{l}\end{array}\right\}$ read the p value from the chart shown on Figure 4.6

$p = 0.013$

Conclusion for plot 2: the null hypothesis is rejected and we consider that the experimental data do not conform to the regression line given by the predicition equation $y = -0.398x + 0.219$.

4.3.1 Pitfalls of the chi-squared test

There are instances when a portion of the regression line yields unrealistic values, whereby the number of calculated nonresponding cultures is larger than the total number of cultures. This is not the case in the above example, but one is discussed in section 4.10.

On the following diagram we depict various possible outcomes of the prediction equations. The legend next to each graph refers to the arrow on the regression line.

In the chi-squared test the amounts of variation present in the set of observation are compared. Small chi-squared values mean small variation and are therefore a better fit.

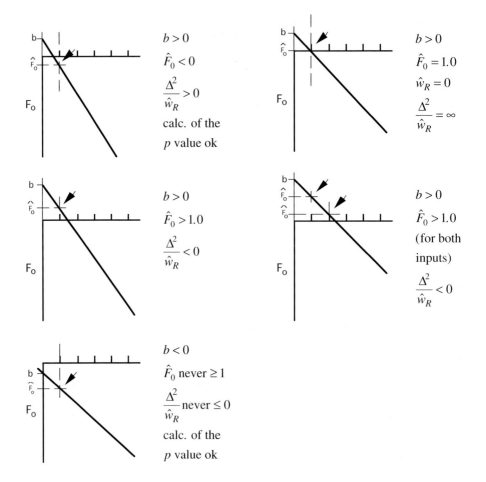

If the prediction equation yields $\hat{w}_R \leq 0$, a calculation of $\dfrac{\Delta^2}{\hat{w}_R}$ should be aborted (the chi-squared sum of the remaining values may be computed but the p value should not be calculated).

4.4   Chi-square-based correlation test

In the previous section we described a chi-squared correlation test for analysing *two sets* of data (observed values vs. calculated values). Here we shall make a small detour and extend the chi-squared test to compare *several sets* of data. We shall abandon the semi-log plotted data and consider a set of micro-cultures whose properties are shown in the following example. Sixty cultures were analysed on eight different plates in order to establish whether there is a correlation between the responding cultures. Thirty-two cultures scored negative on all eight assay plates. Twelve wells were positive on one plate, 7 wells were positive on 2 plates, 3 wells on 3 plates, 4 wells on 4 plates, 1 well was positive on 5 plates, and finally there was also one well which scored positive on all 8 plates. The null hypothesis is that the assays are independent.

The calculation strategy is as follows:

(i)   data are ranked (x, w_x pairs are formed); there will be n lines in the table

        $x = 0, 1, 2 \dots 8$

        w_x = observed number of wells

        $n = k + 1$

        n is the number of data entries, i.e. the number of lines in the evaluation table

        k is the number of assayed plates, each one containing w_T number of wells

(ii)   sum $\left(\Sigma w_x x\right)$ and mean $\left(\dfrac{1}{k}\Sigma w_x x\right)$ are calculated

(iii)   the binomial p is determined as $\dfrac{1}{kw_T}\Sigma w_x x$

(iv)   values $P_0, P_1, P_2, \dots P_k$, are calculated

(v) w_{calc}, the expected number of wells with a given x, is determined

(vi)   values of w_{calc} which are considerably lower than 5 are combined; a new n will result, reflecting the diminished number of entries due to line combining

(vii) $\Delta = \left(w_x - w_{calc}\right)$ is tabulated

(viii) Δ^2 and $\dfrac{\Delta^2}{w_{calc}}$ is computed

        $\left(\dfrac{\Delta^2}{w_{calc}} \text{ are the individual } \chi^2 \text{ contributions}\right)$

(ix)   the total χ^2, i.e. the sum of the individual χ^2 contributions for each x, is calculated as $\chi^2 = \Sigma\dfrac{\Delta^2}{w_{calc}}$

(x)   the number of degrees of freedom ($df = n - 2$) is established

(xi)   the probability value is read from the table

(xii)   the null hypothesis stating that there is no correlation is or is not rejected.

First we prepare a table on which (i) to (v) are dealt with.

Table 4.7. Chi-squared test example

x	w_x	$w_x x$	Binomial for $p = 0.133$	Binomial w_{calc}	
0	32	0	0.318	19.14	
1	12	12	0.392	23.52	
2	7	14	0.211	12.66	
3	3	9	0.065	3.90	< 5
4	4	16	0.012	0.72	< 5
5	1	5	0.002	0.12	< 5
6	0	0	1×10^{-4}	6×10^{-3}	< 5
7	0	0	5×10^{-6}	3×10^{-4}	< 5
$n = k+1 = 9$ 8	1	8	1×10^{-7}	6×10^{-6}	< 5
	60	64	1	60	

Note that $\Sigma w_x x = 64$

and the mean $\dfrac{1}{k}\Sigma w_x x = \dfrac{64}{8} = 8$

The binomial p is $\dfrac{1}{k w_T}\Sigma w_x x = \dfrac{1}{8 \times 60} 64 = 0.133$

Calculation of the binomial distribution values for $p = 0.133, c = 8$.
(N.B. In the binomial formula we keep the letters c and r as derived in Chapter 3, although it would be appropriate to use k and x).

$$P_r = \frac{c!}{r!(c-r)!} p^r q^{c-r}$$

$$P_0 = \frac{8!}{0!\,8!} 0.133^0 \times 0.867^8 = 0.318$$

$$P_1 = \frac{8!}{1!\,7!} 0.133^1 \times 0.867^7 = 0.392$$

etc.

After combining lines 3 – 8 because of the argument (vi) and implementing points (vii – ix) we obtain the following table:

The chi-squared test can be used for comparing observed sets of data with calculated values (section 4.3) or alternatively comparing observed sets of data with values expected from a certain type of probability distribution (section 4.4).

Table 4.8. Chi-squared test example

x	w_x	Binomial for $p = 0.133$	Binomial w_{calc}	$\Delta (w_x - w_{calc})$	Δ^2	$\dfrac{\Delta^2}{w_{calc}}$
0	32	0.319	19.14	12.86	165.38	8.64
1	12	0.392	23.52	11.52	132.71	5.64
2	7	0.211	12.66	5.66	32.04	2.53
$n = 4$ 3	9	0.078	4.68	4.32	18.66	3.99
	60	1	60			20.80

$\chi^2 = 20.80$

$df = n - 2 = 2$

$p = < 0.001$

The chi-squared value $\chi^2 = 20.80$ from the Bliss/Rubes chart (see Appendix and Figure 4.6) gives a probability value $p < 0.001$ for two degrees of freedom. The null hypothesis is rejected and the correlation hypothesis is accepted.

4.5 Test for independence in 2x2 tables

A test of considerable interest in clonal analysis is the test for independence. As with many other tests, we have to be aware of the fact that we can never prove that two events are correlated, but we can accept or reject a hypothesis of independence.

Consider the following experiment. A microculture tray (60 wells) is filled with a spleen cell suspension, antigen X and antigen Y are added, and the cultures are incubated under standard conditions. The culture supernatants are tested on both X and Y indicator cells. We wish to determine whether or not the responses to the two antigens are correlated. So we organise the data in a so-called 2x2 contingency table.

Table 4.9. Box values for the 2x2 table

		Assay X	
		+	−
Assay Y	+	a	b
	−	c	d

Individual values a, b, c, d are referred to as box values. We also include the marginal totals, i.e. the row totals and column totals.

Table 4.10. Row totals and column totals

In order to correlate the probability that a specific set of box values (a, b, c, d) occurs, we need, apart from the null hypothesis, another set of assumptions, to show that the responses are independent. For the purpose of the argument below, we define the 'boundary conditions' so that the marginal totals are fixed. This means that for any given box value, for instance a, the other box values (b, c, d) are determined by the marginal totals; i.e. the probability of the whole set of box values is in fact the probability of only one particular box. Statisticians would say that there is only one degree of freedom associated with the probability. Let us consider a specific example:

Table 4.11. Observed values

The null hypothesis postulates that the results of assays X and Y are independent; the 'expected' 2x2 table based on this hypothesis is calculated as follows:

Fraction of positives in test X	22/60
Fraction of positives in test Y	18/60
Fraction of double positives	$\dfrac{22}{60} \times \dfrac{18}{60}$
Number of double positives	$\dfrac{22}{60} \times \dfrac{18}{60} \times 60 = 6.6$

Are the evaluated two responses independent? We organise the data in a 2x2 contingency table. Fisher's exact probability test allows the hypothesis of independence (section 4.5) to be accepted or rejected.

Table 4.12. Calculated values

		Assay X		
		+	−	
Assay Y	+	6.6	11.4	18
	−	15.4	26.6	42
		22	38	60

Comparing this 'expected' 2x2 table[*] with the experimental one, we realise that the experimental results contain far fewer double positives (3) than expected with the hypothesis of independence (6.6).

The exact probability value associated with our experimental data can be obtained by applying Fisher's exact probability test (Fisher, 1925):

$$f = \frac{(a+b)!\,(c+d)!\,(a+c)!\,(b+d)!}{(a+b+c+d)!} \times \frac{1}{a!\,b!\,c!\,d!}$$

Using the above formula we obtain:

$$f = \frac{18!\,42!\,22!\,38!}{60!} \times \frac{1}{3!\,15!\,19!\,23!}$$

$$f = 0.0258$$

This value of f alone cannot be used to reject the *null hypothesis*. For this we need to know the probability that the present results or *worse* would have been obtained. What do we mean by a *worse* result? Consider the following three results:

Table 4.13. Box values based on fixed marginal totals

2	16	18		1	17	18		0	18	18
20	22	42		21	21	42		22	20	42
22	38	60		22	38	60		22	38	60
f= 0.0056				f= 0.0007				f= 0.00004		

These tables all have the same marginal totals as the experimental results. Clearly they all show a more extreme deviation from the results than would be expected from the hypothesis of independence (the null hypothesis). That is, in

---

[*] Note that the above 2x2 table can be evaluated by the chi-squared test. The calculation is correct when all the values (a_{calc}, b_{calc}, c_{calc}, d_{calc}) are larger than 5. χ^2-approximation would be based on the following calculation:

$$\chi^2 = \frac{(a_{obs} - a_{calc})^2}{a_{calc}} + \frac{(b_{obs} - b_{calc})^2}{b_{calc}} + \frac{(c_{obs} - c_{calc})^2}{c_{calc}} + \frac{(d_{obs} - d_{calc})^2}{d_{calc}}$$

$$df = (2-1)(2-1) = 1$$

every case the value in the upper left hand bar (2, 1, 0) is less than the experimental result (3), which is itself less than would be expected under the null hypothesis (6.6).

Therefore the probability of obtaining the present results is:

$p = 0.0258 + 0.0056 + 0.0007 + 0.00004$

$p = 0.0321$

Should we reject the null hypothesis? At first sight this question seems trivial. Since we agreed at the beginning that we would reject the null hypothesis if the probability of obtaining the results (or worse) was 0.05 or less, and since $p = 0.032$ the case for rejection seems to be straightforward. However, we do so only if we intend to reject the null hypothesis when the two assays X and Y yield too few double positives (the events are anti-correlated). Sometimes this is the case, e.g. when antigenic competition allows a preferential response to one of two test antigens. In general, however, we have no such *a priori* expectation and simply want to know whether the two assays X and Y gave independent results or not. In such a case we would also have rejected the null hypothesis, had there been *too many* (say 18) double positives. Then we would have said that the results of the two assays were correlated (instead of anti-correlated).

Hence we must divide our 'rejection zone' of 5% into two rejection zones of 2.5% each. So we reject the null hypothesis if p calculated for correlation is less than 0.025, or if p calculated for anti-correlation is less than 0.025. In our case clearly we cannot reject the null hypothesis.

The two cases we have discussed here are known conventionally as a one-tailed and a two-tailed test, respectively. The results in the example lead to rejection of the null hypothesis in the one-tailed test and to acceptance in the two-tailed test at the same level of confidence.

Although the calculations performed in this section are simple enough, they are tedious, particularly when the smallest value in the table is greater than 3.

(i) We obtain an experimental set of limiting dilution data and plot the fractions of non-responding cultures against the cell input.

(ii) We establish by linear regression the straight line (through the origin or without constraints of the origin) which fits the data best.

(iii) We evaluate by goodness of fit test whether the line represents a good model (good fit) for the data.

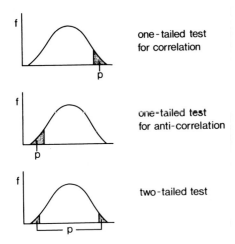

Figure 4.7. One-tailed and two-tailed test.

f, probability value associated with a given set of data; p, the sum of probabilities falling into the 'rejection zone' (shaded area). The curve depicts a normal distribution

In the first edition of this monograph there was a table of the p values for the 2x2 test over 40 pages long. In this edition a complete 2x2 test is included on the diskette accompanying the LDA program.

4.6 Confidence limits of the experimental points

It is obvious that an estimate of the fraction of nonresponding cultures is subject to error. Confidence limits are the most convenient measure of this error. The confidence limits define an interval (in the present case an interval of F_0) with the property that on average in 19 out of 20 cases (95% confidence) or in 99 out of 100 cases (99% confidence) the assumption is correct that the 'true' value (of F_0) falls in that interval.

This interval will be smaller the larger the number of wells used in the assay. In fact, what is meant by the 'true' value is the estimate which would result from an extremely large (conceptually infinitely large) number of wells.

The most frequently used confidence limits by biologists are the 95% confidence limits. These limits are essentially a convention; so much so that many investigators erroneously consider these 95% confidence limits as proof. In Table 4.14 the 95% confidence limits using 60 microcultures are given. A set of tables for other configurations is given in the Appendix to this book.

Table 4.14. Confidence limits as a function of the number of responding cultures for 60 assayed cultures (for other tables see Appendix)

		$w_T = 60$						
w_R	F_0	95% confidence limits		w_R	F_0	95% confidence limits		
		lower	upper			lower		upper
0	1	0.94	–	1				
1	0.98	0.91	–	1	31	0.48	0.35 –	0.62
2	0.97	0.88	–	1	32	0.47	0.34 –	0.60
3	0.95	0.86	–	0.99	33	0.45	0.32 –	0.58
4	0.93	0.84	–	0.98	34	0.43	0.31 –	0.57
5	0.92	0.82	–	0.97	35	0.42	0.29 –	0.55
6	0.90	0.79	–	0.96	36	0.40	0.28 –	0.53
7	0.88	0.77	–	0.95	37	0.38	0.26 –	0.52
8	0.89	0.75	–	0.94	38	0.37	0.25 –	0.50
9	0.85	0.73	–	0.93	39	0.35	0.23 –	0.48
10	0.83	0.71	–	0.92	40	0.33	0.22 –	0.47
11	0.82	0.70	–	0.90	41	0.32	0.20 –	0.45
12	0.80	0.68	–	0.89	42	0.30	0.19 –	0.43
13	0.78	0.66	–	0.88	43	0.28	0.17 –	0.41
14	0.77	0.64	–	0.87	44	0.27	0.16 –	0.40
15	0.75	0.62	–	0.85	45	0.25	0.15 –	0.38
16	0.73	0.60	–	0.84	46	0.23	0.134 –	0.36
17	0.72	0.59	–	0.83	47	0.22	0.120 –	0.34
18	0.70	0.57	–	0.81	48	0.20	0.110 –	0.32
19	0.68	0.55	–	0.80	49	0.18	0.095 –	0.30
20	0.67	0.53	–	0.78	50	0.17	0.083 –	0.29
21	0.65	0.52	–	0.77	51	0.15	0.071 –	0.27
22	0.63	0.50	–	0.75	52	0.133	0.060 –	0.25
23	0.62	0.48	–	0.74	53	0.117	0.048 –	0.23
24	0.60	0.47	–	0.72	54	0.100	0.038 –	0.21
25	0.58	0.45	–	0.71	55	0.083	0.028 –	0.18
26	0.57	0.43	–	0.69	56	0.067	0.018 –	0.16
27	0.55	0.42	–	0.68	57	0.050	0.010 –	0.14
28	0.53	0.40	–	0.66	58	0.033	0.004 –	0.115
29	0.52	0.38	–	0.65	59	0.017	0.001 –	0.089
30	0.50	0.37	–	0.63	60	0	0 –	0.060

In the previous sections of this chapter we dealt with a set of data for which regression lines based on two different models were calculated. We shall now extend our analysis by calculating and plotting the 95% confidence limits of the experimental points.

The lower and upper limits for the above-mentioned data set can be read from Table 4.14. The LDA program with this monograph calculates and displays the 95% confidence limits for various constellations and culture systems.

Table 4.15. Confidence limits of the experimental points. Data from Table 4.1

Cell input			95% confidence limits		
(x 10^{-4} cells/well)	w_R	F_0	lower	–	upper
1	18	0.700	0.57	–	0.81
2	23	0.617	0.48	–	0.74
3	35	0.417	0.29	–	0.55
4	46	0.233	0.134	–	0.36
5	45	0.250	0.15	–	0.38
6	55	0.083	0.028	–	0.18

($w_T = 60$)

The above data plotted on a semi-log scale with 95% confidence limits are as follows:

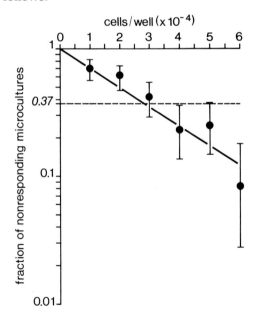

Figure 4.8. 95% confidence limits of the experimental points based upon analysis of sixty culture wells for each of the six tested dilutions

4.7   Confidence limits of the slope

The confidence limits of the experimental points provide useful information on the sampling error of each data point. We shall deal here with yet another confidence limit: one which provides a clue to the reliability of the estimate of the regression line.

The confidence limits of the slope can be conveniently drawn as a shaded area above and below the regression line. The area has a different shape for the regression line forced through the origin and for the line without constraints of the origin, as shown in Figure 4.9.

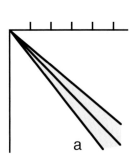

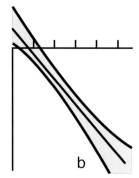

95% confidence fan for a regression line forced through the origin

95% confidence belt for a regression line without constraints of the origin

Figure 4.9. A narrow fan or a narrow belt indicates a good fit to the model, while a wide shaded area suggests that the postulated model might not be a valid one

To establish the confidence limits we use a slightly different procedure for the two regression lines. For the line through the origin ($y = ax$) we calculate the confidence limits a_{upper} and a_{lower} of slope a, and the resulting equations $y = a_{upper} x$, $y = a_{lower} x$ define the boundaries of the fan. For the line not forced through the origin ($y = ax + b$) we calculate the confidence limits for both a and b (a_{upper}, a_{lower}, b_{upper}, b_{lower}). The resulting equations $y = ax + b_{upper}$, $y = ax + b_{lower}$ define the boundaries of the belt (a_{upper}, a_{lower} 'formally' are not present in the equation, but the b term includes the a deviation).

For $y = ax$ the confidence limits $a_{lower} - a_{upper}$ of slope a are calculated from the formula

$$a_{upper} = a + t_{\frac{\alpha}{2}, n-1} \sqrt{\frac{1}{n-1}\left(\frac{\Sigma y_i^2}{\Sigma x_i^2} - a^2\right)}$$

$$a_{lower} = a - t_{\frac{\alpha}{2}, n-1} \sqrt{\frac{1}{n-1}\left(\frac{\Sigma y_i^2}{\Sigma x_i^2} - a^2\right)}$$

Boundary line equations for y_{upper} and y_{lower} $\begin{cases} y = a_{upper}\,x \\ y = a_{lower}\,x \end{cases}$

For $y = ax + b$ the confidence limits $a_{lower} - a_{upper}$ of slope a are calculated from the formula

$$a_{upper} = a + t_{\frac{\alpha}{2}, n-2} \sqrt{\frac{\frac{1}{n-2}\Sigma(y_l - \hat{y}_l)^2}{\Sigma x_i^2 - \frac{1}{n}(\Sigma x_i)^2}}$$

$$a_{lower} = a - t_{\frac{\alpha}{2}, n-2} \sqrt{\frac{\frac{1}{n-2}\Sigma(y_i - \hat{y}_i)^2}{\Sigma x_i^2 - \frac{1}{n}(\Sigma x_i)^2}}$$

The confidence limits of b are given by the formula

$$b_{upper} = b + t_{\frac{\alpha}{2}, n-2} \sqrt{\left(\frac{1}{n-2}\Sigma(y_i - \hat{y}_i)^2\right)\left(\frac{1}{n} + \frac{\left(x - \frac{1}{n}\Sigma x_i\right)^2}{\Sigma x_i^2 - \frac{1}{n}(\Sigma x_i)^2}\right)}$$

$$b_{lower} = b - t_{\frac{\alpha}{2}, n-2} \sqrt{\left(\frac{1}{n-2}\Sigma(y_i - \hat{y}_i)^2\right)\left(\frac{1}{n} + \frac{\left(x - \frac{1}{n}\Sigma x_i\right)^2}{\Sigma x_i^2 - \frac{1}{n}(\Sigma x_i)^2}\right)}$$

Boundary line equations for y_{upper} and y_{lower} $\begin{cases} y = ax + b_{upper} \\ y = ax + b_{lower} \end{cases}$

For the actual calculations we shall use the same set of data which we have dealt with in sections 4.1 and 4.2. We will need the data provided in Table 4.3, though the table displayed on the next page (Table 4.16) is extended by four additional columns (y_i^2, $\hat{y}_i$, $y_i - \hat{y}_i$ and $(y_i - \hat{y}_i)^2$).

Confidence limits of the experimental points provide the measure of error due to the limitation of the number of wells used for a given dilution.

Confidence limits of the slope provide a clue to the reliability of the estimation of the regression line.

Table 4.16. Data for calculating the confidence limits of the slope. Valid for the calculation of the confidence fan ($y = a_{upper}\, x$, $y = a_{lower}\, x$) and the confidence belt ($y = ax + b_{upper}$, $y = ax + b_{lower}$)

	x_i	y_i	$x_i y_i$	x_i^2	y_i^2	$\hat{y}_i$	$y_i - \hat{y}_i$	$(y_i - \hat{y}_i)^2$
	1	− 0.357	− 0.357	1	0.127	− 0.179	− 0.178	0.0317
	2	− 0.483	− 0.967	4	0.234	− 0.577	0.093	0.0087
	3	− 0.876	− 2.626	9	0.766	− 0.975	0.099	0.0099
	4	− 1.455	− 5.821	16	2.118	− 1.373	− 0.083	0.0068
	5	− 1.386	− 6.932	25	1.922	− 1.771	0.384	0.1477
$n = 6$	6	− 2.485	− 14.909	36	6.175	− 2.169	− 0.316	0.1000
	21	− 7.042	− 31.612	91	11.342			0.3048

For the straight line through the origin, $y = ax$, the number of degrees of freedom will be $n - 1$, i.e. 5, while for the straight line without constraints of the origin, $y = ax + b$, the number of degrees of freedom is still one less $n - 2$, i.e. 4. The values for the area α or $\alpha/2$ can be obtained from Student's t-test table (see this page and the Appendix). We mentioned Student in sections 2.4 and 4.3 and more details can be found in the Appendix.

Calculations for $y = -0.347\, x$

$\Sigma y_i^2 = 11.342$

$\Sigma x_i^2 = 91$

$a^2 = (-0.347)^2 = 0.1207$

$df = n - 1 = 5$

$\dfrac{\alpha}{2} = 0.025$

$t_{\frac{\alpha}{2}, n-1} = 2.571$

Table 4.17. Part of Student's t-test table (full table in Appendix).

Degree of freedom	$\dfrac{\alpha}{2} = 0.025$	$\alpha = 0.05$
1	12.706	6.314
2	4.303	2.920
3	3.182	2.353
4	2.776	2.132
5	**2.571**	2.015
6	2.447	1.943
7	2.365	1.895
8	2.306	1.860

The square root term for a

$$\sqrt{\frac{1}{n-1}\left(\frac{\Sigma y_i^2}{\Sigma x_i^2} - a^2\right)} = \sqrt{\frac{1}{5}\left(\frac{11.342}{91} - 0.1207\right)}$$

$$= \sqrt{0.2\,(0.1246 - 0.1207)} = \sqrt{0.00078} = 0.028$$

$a_{upper} = -0.347 + 2.571 \times 0.028 \quad = -0.347 + 0.072 \quad = -0.275$

$a_{lower} = -0.347 - 2.571 \times 0.028 \quad = -0.347 - 0.072 \quad = -0.419$

The boundary equations for the upper and lower limits are
$y = -0.275\,x$ (upper)
$y = -0.419\,x$ (lower)
These confidence limits are depicted in Figure 4.10.

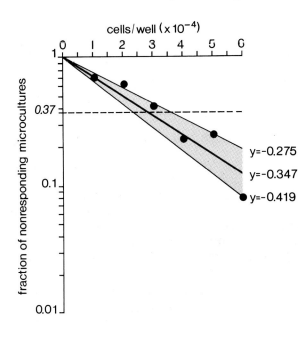

Figure 4.10. 95% confidence limits of the slope (confidence fan) based upon evaluation of the reliability of the regression line estimate (prediction equation through the origin). The upper and lower slope values are obtained from the formula given in the text with the help of Student's t-test table (also see Appendix)

Calculations for $y = -0.398\,x + 0.219$

$\Sigma(y_i - \hat{y}_i)^2 = 0.3048$

$\Sigma x_i^2 = 91$

$\Sigma x_i = 21$

$df = n - 2 = 4$

$\dfrac{\alpha}{2} = 0.025$

$t_{\frac{\alpha}{2},n-2} = 2.776$

Table 4.18. Part of Student's t-test table (full table in Appendix)

Degree of freedom	$\dfrac{\alpha}{2} = 0.025$	$\alpha = 0.05$
1	12.706	6.314
2	4.303	2.920
3	3.182	2.353
4	2.776	2.132
5	2.571	2.015
6	2.447	1.943
7	2.365	1.895
8	2.306	1.860

The square
root term
for b (note
that the
square root
term for a
will not be
needed)

$$\sqrt{\left(\frac{1}{n-2}\Sigma(y_i-\hat{y}_i)^2\right)\left(\frac{1}{n}+\frac{\left(x-\frac{1}{n}\Sigma x_i\right)^2}{\Sigma x_i^2-\frac{1}{n}(\Sigma x_i)^2}\right)} = \sqrt{\left(\frac{1}{6-2}0.3048\right)\left(\frac{1}{6}+\frac{\left(x-\frac{21^2}{6}\right)}{91-\frac{1}{6}(21)^2}\right)}$$

$$= \sqrt{0.0762\left(0.1667+\frac{(x-3.5)^2}{17.5}\right)} = 0.276\sqrt{0.1667+\frac{(x-3.5)^2}{17.5}}$$

$$b_{upper} = 0.219+2.776\times0.276\sqrt{0.1667+\frac{(x-3.5)^2}{17.5}}$$

$$b_{lower} = 0.219-2.776\times0.276\sqrt{0.1667+\frac{(x-3.5)^2}{17.5}}$$

at $x = 0$

$$b_{upper} = 0.219+0.776\sqrt{0.1667+\frac{12.25}{17.5}} = 0.932$$

$$b_{lower} = 0.219-0.776\sqrt{0.1667+0.7} = -0.494$$

The boundary equations for the upper and lower limits are

(upper) $$y = -0.398x+0.219+0.766\sqrt{0.1667+\frac{(x-3.5)^2}{17.5}}$$

(lower) $$y = -0.398x+0.219-0.766\sqrt{0.1667+\frac{(x-3.5)^2}{17.5}}$$

The confidence limits are depicted in Figure 4.11.

We should remember that the prediction equation $y = ax$ allows a simpler interpretation of data than the prediction equation $y = ax + b$, since in a rigorously controlled experiment we do expect Poissonian single-hit kinetics.

Calculating the confidence belt should only be attempted after careful consideration: there is never a problem in the calculation when the value of b is negative, whereas the results of the calculation for positive b are often misleading (see section 4.10).

How many decimal points? One should aim at obtaining end results at a precision which corresponds to 1/10 of standard error. All intermediate calculations should be performed with a precision of an additional 2 decimal points. This is of importance when fractions $\frac{a}{b-c}$ are involved in the calculation and when b and c are large numbers (often of similar magnitude) so that the difference $(b-c)$ is small.

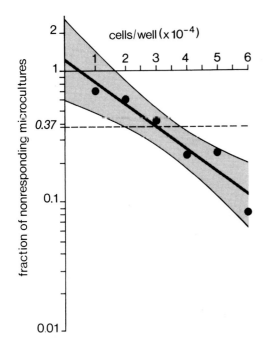

Figure 4.11. 95% confidence limits of the slope (confidence belt) based upon evaluation of the reliability of the regression line estimate (prediction equation without constraints of the origin). The upper and lower slope values are obtained from the formula given in the text with the help of Student's *t*-test table (also see Appendix)

4.8   Maximum likelihood and minimum chi-squared test

Besides the methodology given in the previous sections, there are other approaches for limiting dilution data analysis. Fazekas (1982) suggested the maximum likelihood method, while Taswell (1981, 1987) proposed minimum chi-squared statistics. What both methods have in common is that they are computational rather than graphical, and that the calculations are meaningful only if the experimenter knows that the data conform to a single-hit or another proven model.

4.8.1   Maximum likelihood test

Data from a limiting dilution assay are submitted to calculation in two steps:

   (i)   calculation of a provisional value of $1/f$ is performed

   (ii) iterative solution of the maximum likelihood equation by the Finney routine (Finney, 1951) is achieved in several cycles. The results of each cycle are the provisional estimates for the next cycle until the improvement to the previous estimate is negligible.

It is convenient to illustrate the maximum likelihood method with the example already shown in sections 4.1, 4.3 and 4.7, since Fazekas used our example in his 1982 paper to illustrate the suggested procedure.

Table 4.19. Maximum likelihood method

x (x 10^{-4} cells/well)	w_R	F_0	$\ln F_0$	$\ln(-\ln F_0)$	$\ln x$	$\ln(-\ln F_0) - \ln x$
1	18	0.7	− 0.357	− 1.031	0	− 1.031
2	23	0.62	− 0.483	− 0.727	0.693	− 1.420
3	35	0.42	− 0.876	− 0.133	1.099	− 1.232
4	46	0.23	− 1.455	0.375	1.386	− 1.011
5	45	0.25	− 1.386	0.327	1.609	− 1.282
6	55	0.083	− 2.485	0.910	1.792	− 0.882
					sum	− 6.858
					mean	− 1.143

Cell dose containing 1 precursor cell: anti-log −1.143   3.1361
multiplied by 10^4 = 31361 cells

The value −1.143 is then plugged into the iterative maximum likelihood equation using a routine devised by Finney (1951). The solution is obtained in 3 successive cycles:

Table 4.20. Iteration (3 cycles)

Cycle	Cell dose (1/f)	ln (1/f)
1	3.1361 (x 10^4)	1.143
2	3.1425 (x 10^4)	1.14502
3	3.1426 (x 10^4)	1.14505

Solution: $1/f$ = 31426 cells, f = 3.18 x 10^{-5}
95% conf. limits: 27285 – 36194 cells
χ^2 = 5.767
p = 0.329

The χ^2 results (and p values) were taken directly from Fazekas (1982).

Further details on the maximum likelihood method will be given on the website.

The reader should compare the above data with those obtained in sections 4.1, 4.3 and 4.7.

Note that the model which Finney originally developed for situations in which binomially distributed samples are assumed was further developed by Nelder and Wedderburn (1972) into a so-called 'generalised linear model'. In essence, Nelder extended Finney's model for situations in which wide families of distributions (normal, Poisson, gamma) are considered.

4.8.2   Chi-squared minimisation test

Taswell's procedure (1987) is a computational method performed in two steps.

(i)   A test is performed to establish that the data conform to a single-hit Poisson model. The regression slope test (degrees of freedom = 1) is performed, and if the single-hit model is not rejected the data are submitted to the actual minimum chi-squared test.

(ii)   The minimum chi-squared frequency estimate is calculated as the value of frequency that minimises Pearson's chi-square (χ^2) by Newton's method of iterative approximation using the first and second partial derivatives of χ^2.

Neither the maximum likelihood test nor the minimum chi-squared estimates are implemented in the present version of the accompanying LDA software, though these procedures will be included in later versions. The pros and cons for using the maximum likelihood test and the minimum chi-squared test are given in section 4.9.

4.9   Critical appraisal

It might be of more than just historical interest to recall that in the eighties there was a heated debate on the use of various statistical methods for obtaining 'better' frequency estimates. We argued (Lefkovits and Waldmann, 1984) that it does not matter which method is used to estimate the μ parameter, since the resulting estimate represents an approximate assessment of biological activity and not an absolutely precise determination of a physical constant. Taswell (1987) pointed out that 'although it is certainly true that physico-chemical parameters can be measured more accurately and precisely than biological procedures, this fact does not justify avoiding measuring biological parameters as accurately as possible'.

Taswell's statement is such a truism that we can do no better than endorse it. Still, we think that striving for a 'better' and 'more precise' estimate might provide the experimenter with a false feeling of getting adequate results without scrutinising the methodology of statistics.

We suggest that interested readers get acquainted with Taswell's excellent review (1987) and with the papers of Berkson (1980) and Fazekas (1982). The title of Berkson's paper indicates that the debate was without compromise: 'Minimum chi-square, not maximum likelihood!'. The paper of Fazekas contains an interesting proposition on the 'most informative range' (see section

5.3), and a description of the procedure for obtaining frequency estimates using the maximum likelihood test. Below we show that the procedure yields 'precise' results, but that they are of limited usefulness and certainly do not offer an attractive alternative to the procedures listed in sections 4.1 and 4.2.

The frequency estimates obtained with three different procedures and based on one and the same data set – dealt with in sections 4.1, 4.2 and 4.8 – are summarised below.

Table 4.21. The single-hit model yields identical results both by calculation from the prediction equation $y = -0.347\ x$ and by reading the 37% intercept (28 800 cells). Models based on some kind of cooperativity (see under targetness) with a prediction equation $y = -0.398\ x + 0.219$ yield a cell dose value of 25 063. The 37% intercept is incorrect, while the reading of slope at ∆ 37% is correct yielding about ∆ 25 000 cells

Method of analysis	Frequency estimate (f)	Cell dose containing 1 prec. cell ($1/f$)	Intercept with 37% line	
			x value	note
Linear regression through the origin	3.47×10^{-5}	28818	28800	correct (slope through the origin)
Linear regression disregarding the origin	3.98×10^{-5}	25063	30700	incorrect (intercept meaningless)
Maximum likelihood test	3.18×10^{-5}	31426		

Fazekas' maximum likelihood calculations yield an estimate (31 426 cells), which is similar to a value which we would obtain by an incorrect procedure of reading the 37% intercept in Figure 4.3. Differences in the results using different procedures of calculation should sensitise the reader to judging the results cautiously and critically.

In conclusion, the statistical methods described in this chapter aim at obtaining consistent and reliable information on various parameters of LDA. To do this, we rely heavily on the graphical representation of the results. The semi-log plot is uniquely suited to enhance our visual capability to interpret the results, to judge whether the conditions of single-hit kinetics are maintained and, as a gratuitous side product of this approach, the frequency estimate can be read directly from the graph.

Taswell distinguishes between 'computational' and 'graphical' methods. His procedure (and that of Fazekas) is a computational technique which is '*readily amenable to graphical presentation for investigators who so desire, though they should draw their conclusions from values of test statistics and not from appearance of graphs*' (Taswell, 1987). We do not share this attitude as it is our long-standing experience that limiting dilution data without graphical presentation (in the form of semi-log plots) are quite incomplete and imperfect.

4.10   An exercise

We have dealt with linear regression, goodness of fit, confidence limits (experimental points/slope) using real data (sections 4.1–4.3, 4.6, 4.7) on a B-cell titration. We will repeat all these steps, but with data from another B-cell titration.

Table 4.22. Results of a B-cell titration (second example)

x_i (x 10^{-4} cells/well)	y_i		
	w_R	F_0	$\ln F_0$
1	0	1	0
2	3	0.95	− 0.051
3	24	0.60	− 0.511
4	54	0.10	− 2.302

$(w_T = 60)$

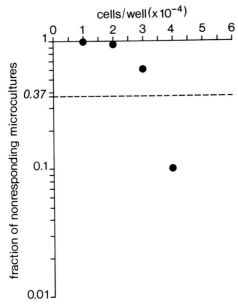

Figure 4.12. Experimental data of a B-cell titration displayed on a semi-log scale (although clearly not single-hit kinetics, it will be treated as if it were)

We shall derive the prediction equation for the least square linear regression line through the origin. We shall calculate a for the function $y = ax$.

$$a = \frac{\Sigma x_i y_i}{\Sigma x_i^2}$$

The above set of data can be rearranged so that $\Sigma x_i y_i$ and Σx_i^2 are the sums of the data columns.

Table 4.23. Data for calculating the regression line

	x_i	y_i	$x_i y_i$	x_i^2
	1	0	0	1
	2	− 0.051	− 0.103	4
	3	− 0.511	− 1.532	9
$n = 4$	4	− 2.302	− 9.210	16
	10	− 2.864	− 10.845	30

$$a = \frac{\Sigma x_i y_i}{\Sigma x_i^2} = \frac{-10.845}{30} = -0.362$$

$$y = -0.362\, x$$

Frequency estimate ($\times 10^4$) $= 0.362$

Frequency estimate $\quad f = 0.362 \times 10^{-4}$

$$= 3.62 \times 10^{-5}$$

$$\frac{1}{f} = \frac{1}{3.62 \times 10^{-5}} = 27\,600 \text{ cells}$$

cell dose containing 1 precursor cell on average

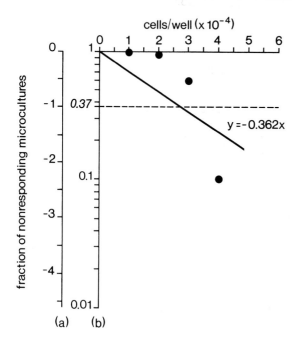

Figure 4.13. Fitting straight line through the origin. The straight line was fitted by the method of least squares; linear function $y = -0.362\, x$ was converted for plotting into a logarithmic one. a) Logarithmic values on a linear scale; b) Linear values on a logarithmic scale

We shall derive the prediction equation for the least square regression line disregarding the origin.

$$\Sigma x_i y_i = -10.845$$

$$\Sigma x_i = 10$$

$$\Sigma y_i = -2.864$$

$$\Sigma x_i^2 = 30$$

$$n = 4$$

We shall find a and b for the fraction $y = ax + b$.

$$a = \frac{n\Sigma x_i y_i - (\Sigma x_i)(\Sigma y_i)}{n\Sigma x_i^2 - (\Sigma x_i)^2} = -\frac{4 \times 10.845 - 10 \times 2.864}{4 \times 30 - 10 \times 10} = -0.736$$

$$b = \bar{y} - a\bar{x} = \left(\frac{\Sigma y_i}{n}\right) - a\left(\frac{\Sigma x_i}{n}\right) = -\frac{2.864}{4} + 0.736\frac{10}{4} = 1.125$$

$$y = -0.736\, x + 1.125$$

Values for the slope and the y intercept converted to F_0 are as follows:

for $a = -0.736$ F_0 is 0.479

for $b = 1.125$ F_0 is 3.08

Frequency estimate (x 10^4)   = 0.736

Frequency estimate f = 0.736 x 10^{-4}

= 7.36 x 10^{-5}

$$\frac{1}{f} = \frac{1}{7.36 \times 10^{-5}} = 13\,600 \text{ cells}$$

cell dose containing 1 precursor cell on average

The y axis can be considered for convenience in two forms (as indicated in Figures 4.2 and 4.3). In one we can plot logarithmic values on a linear scale, in the other, linear values on a logarithmic scale.

The so-called 37% line intercepts the linear scale at a value of -1.

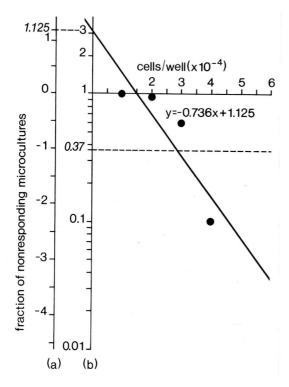

(a)　(b)

Figure 4.14. Fitting a straight line without the constraints of the origin. a) Logarithmic values on a linear scale. b) Linear values on a logarithmic scale

We continue to evaluate the goodness of fit of the experimental points to both prediction equations:

$$y = -0.362\,x \qquad\qquad \text{and} \qquad\qquad y = -0.736\,x + 1.125.$$

The number of responding (or nonresponding) wells expected from the prediction equation(s) is calculated.

Table 4.24. Tabulated values calculated from the prediction equations

	$y = -0.362\,x$				$y = -0.736\,x + 1.125$		
x	y	$\hat{F}_0$	$\hat{w}_- = 60 \times \hat{F}_0$	x	y	$\hat{F}_0$	$\hat{w}_- = 60 \times \hat{F}_0$
1	−0.362	0.697	41.80	1	0.389	1.475	88.52
2	−0.723	0.485	29.12	2	−0.348	0.706	42.37
3	−1.085	0.338	20.28	3	−1.085	0.338	20.28
4	−1.446	0.235	14.13	4	−1.821	0.162	9.71

Warning: the prediction equation $y = -0.736\,x + 1.125$ yielded an unrealistic value of 88.52 nonresponding cultures (since $F_0 > 1$); this will be omitted from χ^2 calculations. Note that 88.52 nonresponding cultures mean −28.52 responding cultures

For the above two approaches we postulate the null hypotheses:

(i) the experimental data conform to single-hit kinetics ($y = -0.362 x$)

(ii) the experimental data conform to the regression line without constraints of the origin ($y = -0.736 x + 1.125$).

The goodness of fit of the experimental points to the prediction equation $y = -0.362 x$ is calculated as follows:

Table 4.25. Display of the tabulated values for χ^2 calculations (through the origin)

x_i	$y_{i(obs)}$		$\hat{y}_{i(calc)}$		Δw	Δ^2	$\dfrac{\Delta^2}{\hat{w}_R}$	$\dfrac{\Delta^2}{\hat{w}_-}$
	w_R	w_-	$\hat{w}_R$	$\hat{w}_-$				
1	0	60	18.20	41.80	18.20	331.3	18.2	7.9
2	3	57	30.88	29.12	27.88	777.5	25.2	26.7
3	24	36	39.72	20.28	15.72	247.0	6.2	12.2
4	54	6	45.87	14.13	8.13	66.1	1.5	4.7
							51.1	51.5

$\chi^2 = 51.1 + 51.5 = 102.6$ } read the p value from the Bliss/Rubes
$df = n - 1 = 3$ chart in the Appendix
$p < 0.001$

The null hypothesis is rejected and the experimental data are considered not to conform to single-hit kinetics.

The goodness of fit of the experimental points to the prediction equation $y = -0.736x + 1.125$ (line without constraints of the origin) is calculated as follows:

Table 4.26. Display of the tabulated values for χ^2 calculations (disregarding the origin)

	x_i	$y_{i(obs)}$		$\hat{y}_{i(calc)}$		Δw	Δ^2	$\dfrac{\Delta^2}{\hat{w}_R}$	$\dfrac{\Delta^2}{\hat{w}_-}$
		w_R	w_-	$\hat{w}_R$	$\hat{w}_-$				
	1	0	60	-28.52	88.52	omitted from calculation			
	2	3	57	17.63	42.37	14.63	213.9	12.1	5.0
	3	24	36	39.72	20.28	15.72	247.0	6.2	12.2
$n = 4$	4	54	6	50.29	9.71	3.71	13.8	0.3	1.4
								18.6	18.6

$\chi^2 = 37.2$

$df = (n-1) - 2 = 1$

Warning: the p value should not be calculated

The null hypothesis is not tested. Incidentally, if we opt for a more permissive approach and test the hypothesis, it is rejected ($p < 0.001$, Appendix) and the experimental data are considered not to conform to the prediction equation $y = -0.736x + 1.125$. In the LDA program (Chapter 10) we have chosen another approach whereby the contribution of the values based on $\hat{w}_R < 0$ is omitted, but the p value is calculated from the remaining χ^2 terms.

Neither the straight line through the origin, nor the one without constraints of the origin, can be considered as usable for describing the results as single-hit events (or multi-target events based on a 'definite slope').

4.10.1 95% confidence limits

95% confidence limits of the experimental points are read from Table 4.14.

Table 4.27. Confidence limits of the experimental points. Data from Table 4.22

| Cell input | | | 95% confidence limits | |
(x 10^{-4} cells/well)	w_R	F_0	lower –	upper
1	0	1	0.94 –	1
2	3	0.95	0.86 –	0.99
3	24	0.60	0.47 –	0.72
4	54	0.10	0.038 –	0.21

($w_T = 60$)

The above data plotted on a semi-log scale with 95% confidence limits are:

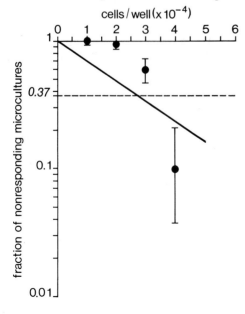

Figure 4.15. 95% confidence limits of the experimental points based upon analysis of sixty culture wells for each of the six tested dilutions

4.10.2 Confidence limits of the slope

Formulae for the confidence fan and the confidence belt:

Confidence fan for $y = ax$

$$a_{upper/lower} = a \pm t_{\frac{\alpha}{2}, n-1} \sqrt{\frac{1}{n-1}\left(\frac{\Sigma y_i^2}{\Sigma x_i^2} - a^2\right)}$$

$$y = a_{upper}x$$

$$y = a_{lower}x$$

Confidence belt for $y = ax + b$

$$a_{upper/lower} = a \pm t_{\frac{\alpha}{2}, n-2} \sqrt{\frac{\frac{1}{n-2}\Sigma(y_i - \hat{y}_i)^2}{\Sigma x_i^2 - \frac{1}{n}\left(\Sigma x_i^2\right)^2}}$$

$$b_{upper/lower} = b \pm t_{\frac{\alpha}{2}, n-2} \sqrt{\left(\frac{1}{n-2}\Sigma(y_i - \hat{y}_i)^2\right)\left(\frac{1}{n} + \frac{\left(x - \frac{1}{n}\Sigma x_i\right)^2}{\Sigma x_i^2 - \frac{1}{n}\left(\Sigma x_i\right)^2}\right)}$$

$$y = ax + b_{upper}$$

$$y = ax + b_{lower}$$

We shall use the data from Table 4.23 extended by columns y_i^2, $\hat{y}_i$, $y_i - \hat{y}_i$ and $\left(y_i - \hat{y}_i\right)^2$

Table 4.28. Data for calculating the confidence limits of the slope. Valid for the calculation of the confidence fan ($y = a_{upper}\,x$, $y = a_{lower}\,x$) and the confidence belt ($y = ax + b_{upper}$, $y = ax + b_{lower}$)

	x_i	y_i	$x_i y_i$	x_i^2	y_i^2	$\hat{y}_i$	$y_i - \hat{y}_i$	$\left(y_i - \hat{y}_i\right)^2$
	1	0	0	1	0	− 0.389	− 0.389	0.1513
	2	− 0.051	− 0.103	4	0.003	− 0.348	0.2967	0.0880
	3	− 0.511	− 1.532	9	0.26	− 1.085	0.5742	0.3297
$n = 4$	4	− 2.302	− 9.210	16	5.29	− 1.821	− 0.4816	0.2319
	10	− 2.864	− 10.845	30	5.553			0.8009

Calculations for $y = -0.362\,x$

Table 4.29. Part of Student's *t*-test table
(full table in Appendix)

Degree of freedom	$\dfrac{\alpha}{2} = 0.025$	$\alpha = 0.05$
1	12.706	6.314
2	4.303	2.920
3	**3.182**	2.353
4	2.776	2.132
5	2.571	2.015
6	2.447	1.943
7	2.365	1.895
8	2.306	1.860

$\Sigma y_i^2 = 5.553$

$\Sigma x_i^2 = 30$

$a^2 = (-0.362)^2 = 0.1310$

$df = n - 1 = 3$

$\dfrac{\alpha}{2} = 0.025$

$t_{\frac{\alpha}{2}, n-1} = 3.182$

The square root term for a:
$$\sqrt{\frac{1}{n-1}\left(\frac{\Sigma y_i^2}{\Sigma x_i^2} - a^2\right)} = \sqrt{\frac{1}{3}\left(\frac{5.553}{30} - (0.362)^2\right)}$$

$$= \sqrt{0.333\,(0.1851 - 0.1310)} = \sqrt{0.01803} = 0.134$$

$a_{upper} = -0.362 + 3.182 \times 0.134 = 0.071$
$a_{lower} = -0.398 - 3.182 \times 0.134 = -0.795$

The boundary equations for the upper and lower limits are
$y = 0.071\,x$ (upper)
$y = -0.795\,x$ (lower)
These confidence limits of the slope are depicted in Figure 4.16.

Degrees of freedom
The term degrees of freedom (df) refers to the number of independent samples. The number of degrees of freedom equals in most instances n-1, where n is the sample size.

Just as there are many normal distributions, there are also many t-distributions and chi-square distributions. For df > 30 both t- and χ^2-distributions can be approximated by the normal distribution.

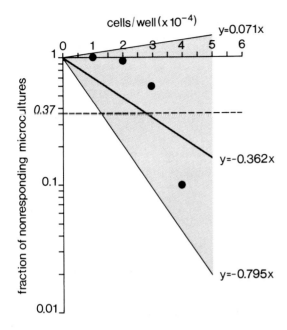

Figure 4.16. 95% confidence limits of the slope (confidence fan) based upon evaluation of the reliability of the regression line estimate (prediction equation through the origin). The upper and lower slope values are obtained from the formula given in the text with the help of Student's t-test table (see also Appendix)

Calculations for $y = -0.736\,x + 1.125$

$\Sigma(y_i - \hat{y}_i)^2 = 0.8009$

$\Sigma x_i^2 = 30$

$df = n - 2 = 1$

$\dfrac{\alpha}{2} = 0.025$

$t_{\frac{\alpha}{2},n-1} = 12.706$

Table 4.30. Part of Student's t-test table (full table in Appendix).

Degree of freedom	$\dfrac{\alpha}{2} = 0.025$	$\alpha = 0.05$
1	**12.706**	6.314
2	4.303	2.920
3	3.182	2.353
4	2.776	2.132
5	2.571	2.015
6	2.447	1.943
7	2.365	1.895
8	2.306	1.860

The square root term for b:

$$\sqrt{\left(\frac{1}{n-2}\right)\frac{1}{h}\left(\frac{x-\frac{1}{n}\Sigma y_i^2}{\Sigma x_i^2-\frac{1}{n}\left(\Sigma x_i\right)^2}\right)} = \sqrt{\left(\frac{1}{4-2}0.8009\right)\left(\frac{1}{4}+\frac{\left(x-\frac{10}{4}\right)^2}{30-\frac{1}{4}\times 10^2}\right)}$$

$$=\sqrt{0.5\times 0.8009\left(0.25+\frac{(x-2.5)^2}{5}\right)}=0.633\sqrt{0.25+\frac{(x-2.5)^2}{5}}$$

$$b_{upper}=1.125+12.706\times 0.633\sqrt{0.25+\frac{(x-2.5)^2}{5}}$$

$$b_{lower}=1.125-12.706\times 0.633\sqrt{0.25+\frac{(x-2.5)^2}{5}}$$

at $x=0$ $$b_{upper}=1.125+8.043\sqrt{0.25+\frac{6.25}{5}}=4.460$$

$$b_{lower}=1.125-8.043\sqrt{0.25+\frac{6.25}{5}}=2.210$$

The boundary equations for the upper and lower limits are

$$y=-0.736x+1.125+8.043\sqrt{0.25+\frac{(x-2.5)^2}{5}}$$

$$y=-0.736x+1.125-8.043\sqrt{0.25+\frac{(x-2.5)^2}{5}}$$

The boundaries given by the two equations are so 'wide' that they cannot be depicted on the scale of our semi-log plot. For didactic purposes we depict in Figure 4.17 the confidence limits for the equation pair which utilises $df = 2$, and $\alpha/2 = 4.303$.
The equations are

$$y=-0.736x+1.125+2.723\sqrt{0.25+\frac{(x-2.5)^2}{5}}$$

$$y=-0.736x+1.125-2.723\sqrt{0.25+\frac{(x-2.5)^2}{5}}$$

y intercept. Multi-target curves have a definite slope, which extrapolated to the y axis is a measure for the number of cell categories required for eliciting a response (multi-hit curves [section 5.5] are concave; no definite slope).

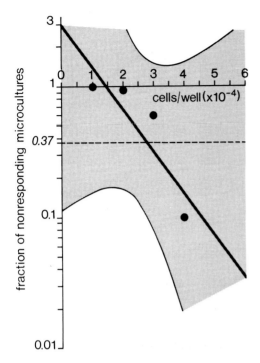

Figure 4.17. 95% confidence limits of the slope. The shaded area above the *x* axis is not interpretable; this provides another indication that the data cannot be explained by single-hit models. Note that the belt is based on $df = 2$ ($\alpha/2 = 4.303$)

4.11 Summary of examples

In the ten pictograms on the next page we summarise the most important features of the procedures described in this chapter.

The plots are based on two sets of data (Tables 4.1. and 4.22). The left block refers to the procedure given in sections 4.1, 4.2, 4.6 and 4.7, while the right block summarises the data and the calculations given in section 4.10.

Note that the pictogram in the second row refers to the procedure for calculating the confidence limits of the experimental points, while the bottom row depicts the confidence limits of the slope.

The experimental data of the left block fulfil the criteria of a single-hit model. The experimental data of the right block are interpreted as multi-hit titrations.

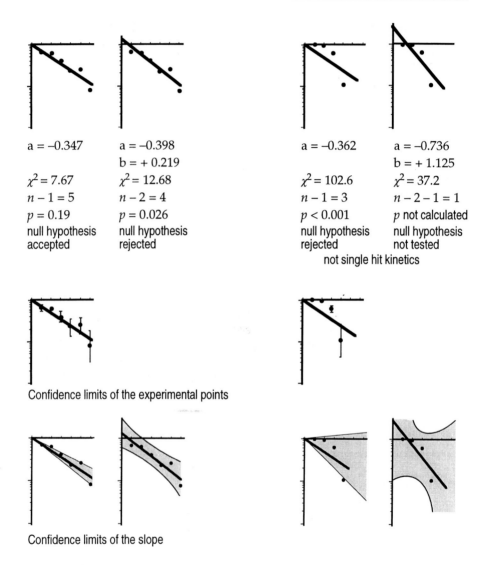

Figure 4.18. Linear regression through the origin, without constraints of the origin, chi-squared test for goodness of fit, confidence limits of experimental points and confidence limits of the slope

5   Models of limiting dilution analysis

In previous chapters we dealt with theoretical aspects of the Poissonian processes and basic considerations for statistical analysis. Here we will consider ways to analyse single and multi-hit events, to distinguish between hittedness and targetness, and we will cover several other concepts of limiting dilution. We will learn to identify and interpret different forms of titration curves. However, we will *not* deal with the analysis of cellular interactions as we have reserved Chapter 6 for that.

5.1   Dilutions

Poissonian analysis of cells can be performed at one or several cell doses. In some instances the experiments based on one cell input yield valid results, in others the use of several cell inputs is a prerequisite for correctly interpreting the results.

Let us examine two experimental situations:

(i)   the cells in the analysed population do not require anything other than an antigenic signal to elicit a measurable antibody response;

(ii)   the cells in the analysed population require other signals (cell interactions, etc.) besides the antigenic signal

We will now consider the results obtained from culturing many small aliquots of lymphocytes in the presence of antigen. At the end of the culture period we will be able to identify a certain portion of responding cultures. In the experimental situation (i) a lack of response will be expected only in those samples where antigen-specific precursor cells are missing; in the experimental situation (ii) there might be wells which contain precursor cells which in fact had the capability to respond to the antigen but were prevented from eliciting a response because 'other required cell types' were missing.

Clearly, in situation (i) the observed fraction of nonresponding samples is a valid clue for estimating the mean number of precursor cells (μ) per sample. In situation (ii) the calculation will yield an underestimated value of μ since some precursor cells in the population remained undetected.

How would the analysis change if in both experimental situations we apply several different cell inputs? In situation (i) we obtain results which upon plotting in a semi-log fashion will reveal that the process is indeed based on single-hit kinetics and that a valid frequency estimate can be read at the 37% intercept. In an ideal case this estimate would be very similar to the one obtained by computing the frequency from the *fraction of nonresponding cultures* observed at a single-cell dilution.

In situation (ii) the semi-log plot might fit to a straight line or will deviate from it significantly depending on whether or not there was an excess of other required cell types.

As will be explained in detail later, the plot can be used to interpret the results, to recognise the need for complementing the cell population with other required cells and, finally, to obtain valid frequency estimates.

The expressions 'cell input', 'cell dose' and 'dilutions' are used synonymously. Obviously, in cases when we work with 'one cell input' we refrain from using the word 'dilution', since by dilution we are implying that there are several cell inputs.

5.2   Cells limiting, cells in excess

Limiting dilution analysis is based on culturing many small aliquots of cells. The aliquots must be of such a size that the cells of interest are present in some and absent in others. There are two extreme situations which are useless for analysis: one is when the aliquots are so small (so diluted) that the measured set yields no positive cultures, the other is when the aliquots are so large (so dense) that all cultures become positive. It is convenient to choose several dilutions which lie in between. Such an arrangement meets the requirement for the presence/absence of the measured cell type in a portion of the cultures. Another requirement is that all other components – whether molecular or cellular in nature – are present in excess. 'Excess', in fact, is not the right word, since what is meant is that in each well there should be 'enough' of all the required components (except the measured one). The word excess does not catch this meaning fully, as excess might be 'too much'. We often say that other components have to be present in *saturating* amounts (molecules) or numbers (cells).

The semi-log plot implies that the experiment is planned and executed so that the cell input covers a linear range (experimental points more or less equidistantly spaced). For a preliminary experiment one chooses a broad range of dilutions, and from the results one identifies the proper linear range – as indicated in Figure 5.1.

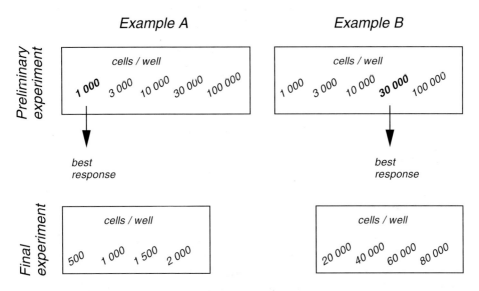

Figure 5.1. Choice of cell dilutions for the preliminary experiment (wide range) and the final experiment (linear range)

We should be aware of the fact that in order to achieve comparable culture conditions for all cell inputs, the cell density should be maintained constant by adding so-called filler cells. Filler cells do not participate in the response but create the proper conditions for growth, differentiation and response to take place. If the cell density for the culture is envisaged at 100 000 cells/well, the filler cell input for the above five dilutions of the preliminary experiment (Figure 5.1) should be 99 000, 97 000, 90 000, 70 000, nil. Details on filler cells will be given in Chapter 7.

5.3 Informative range

Mather (1949) and Fazekas (1982) recognised that the results of quantal responses at the two extremes (very low and very high F_0) are less robust, less reliable, or, in Mather's definition, contain 'less information per unit observation', than when F_0 is of intermediate value. The amount of information is the weighting coefficient, which can be plotted against the p value. Figure 5.1 reproduces Mather's curve. According to Fazekas (1982) the highest information content is achieved with a cell input where the multiplicity of 1.59 can be expected.

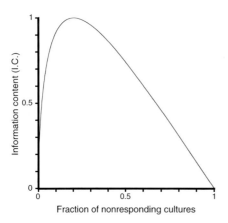

Figure 5.2. Information content (I.C.) plotted
against the fraction of nonresponding cultures

What is the take-home lesson from the concept of the 'most informative range'? Should we abandon the notion of applying an equidistant linear range of dilutions, and should we concentrate on the region with the highest information content? Or, alternatively, should we stick to the linear range but vary the number of cultures per experimental point (e.g. use a large number of cultures where a high information content is expected)?

The answer is neither/nor. Although the aim of LD experiments is to estimate the frequency of cells involved in the response, the conditions for single-hit kinetics have to be monitored. To ensure that the frequency can be estimated correctly, we should use a protocol which allows both the single-hit monitoring and reliable experimental readout – this is best achieved using a linear range of the cell inputs and choosing equal numbers of cultures for all the experimental points.

Note that an extreme proposition from the informative range would be to choose only a single dilution at an input where a multiplicity of 1.59 is expected and perform as many cultures as possible at that dilution. This would still be a good Poissonian analysis but certainly not a limiting dilution analysis.

5.4   Single-hit events

For readers who have bypassed the theory chapter, we will briefly summarise the rationale for using the semi-log plot and we will explain the basis of single-hit events.

From the zero term of the Poisson distribution ($F_0 = e^{-\mu}$) and its logarithmic form ($\mu = -\ln F_0$) we can state that the negative logarithm of the fraction of nonresponding cultures is linearly proportional to the mean number of precursor cells per culture.

It follows that if we plot on the y axis the negative logarithm of the fraction of nonresponding cultures ($-\ln F_0$) and the cell input on the linear scale on the x axis, we expect the experimental points to fit a straight line passing through the origin. Further, the semi-log plot is a convenient way to estimate the frequency of precursor cells, because by interpolating at the level of 37% nonresponding cultures, the size of the sample containing an average of one precursor cell can be directly estimated (Figure 5.3).

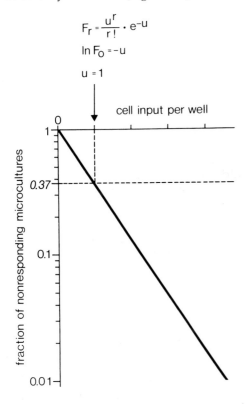

$$F_r = \frac{u^r}{r!} \cdot e^{-u}$$

$$\ln F_0 = -u$$

$$u = 1$$

cell input per well

fraction of nonresponding microcultures

1

0.37

0.1

0.01

Figure 5.3. Semi-log plot

At this point it has to be stressed that the single-hit curve is compatible with the hypothesis that we are dealing with a single cell type dilution, but it is not proof of it.

In summary, the fraction of nonresponding cultures decreases exponentially as the number of precursor cells is increased, and the linearity in the semi-log plot (single-hit curve) supports the hypothesis that only a single-cell type is being diluted out. Thirty-seven per cent of nonresponding cultures should be expected when there is a mean of one precursor cell per culture.

5.5   Multi-hit model

Target and hit theories have been formulated by Dessauer (1922), Blau and Altenburger (1922) and Crowther (1924) for explaining the effects of ionising radiation on living cells. Adopting the target and hit theories for the limiting dilution analysis in the immune system, we make the following definition:

> a multi-hit model might explain the experimental results when a measurable antibody response is only elicited if at least n cells are present in the sample.

We have only one category of cells, and the only samples that will respond are those containing at least n cells. All the following fractions of samples have less than n cells:

$$e^{-\mu}, \mu e^{-\mu}, \frac{\mu^2}{2!}e^{-\mu}, \cdots, \frac{\mu^{n-1}}{(n-1)!}e^{-\mu}$$

$$0 \quad\quad 1 \quad\quad 2 \quad\quad\quad\quad n-1$$

and the sum of these fractions constitutes the nonresponding cultures (Figure 5.4):

$$F_0 = e^{-\mu} + \mu e^{-\mu} + \frac{\mu^2}{2!}e^{-\mu} + \cdots + \frac{\mu^{n-1}}{(n-1)!}e^{-\mu}$$

$$F_0 = \left(1 + \mu + \frac{\mu^2}{2} + \cdots + \frac{\mu^{n-1}}{(n-1)!}\right)e^{-\mu}$$

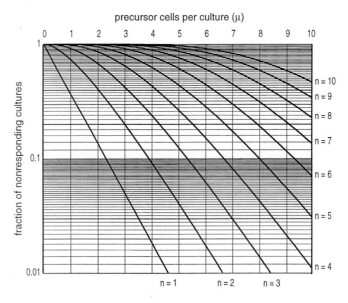

Figure 5.4. Multi-hit model (*n* cells)

5.6   Multi-target model

The multi-target model is defined as follows:

a measurable antibody response is elicited only if at least one cell of each of the m categories is present in the sample.

The fraction of samples containing one or more cells of one category	$1-e^{-\mu}$
The fraction of samples containing one or more cells of m categories	$\left(1-e^{-\mu}\right)^{m}$
The fraction of nonresponding cultures (missing at least one of the m categories)	$F_0 = 1-\left(1-e^{-\mu}\right)^{m}$

Note that the semi-log plot of the multi-target curve has a definite slope, which extrapolated to the y axis is a measure for the number of targets (number of cell categories) required for eliciting a response (Figure 5.5). This is not the case for a multi-hit curve where the curve remains concave and does not assume a definite slope (Figure 5.4).

The above formula for a multi-target event is only correct if the size of each category is the same, i.e. the ratio is 1:1. If the ratio is different from 1:1, the equation is more complex.

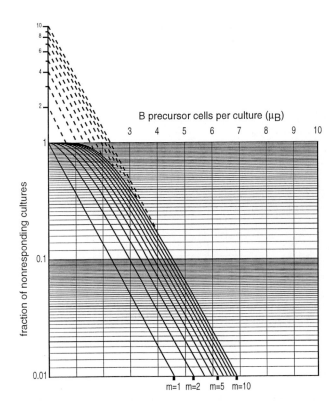

Figure 5.5. Multi-target model (*m* categories of cells). Extrapolation to *y* axis

Now we will show a relatively simple case of a two-cell cooperation (B and T), where the ratio of the two cell types varies. A measurable response is elicited if at least one B cell and one T cell is present in the sample:

$$F_0 = 1 - \left(1 - e^{-\mu_B}\right)\left(1 - e^{-\mu_T}\right)$$

$$F_0 = e^{-\mu_B} + e^{-\mu_T} - e^{-(\mu_B + \mu_T)}$$

We assume a ratio of T to B cells = a

$$\frac{\mu_T}{\mu_B} = a$$

$$\mu_T = a\mu_B$$

$$F_0 = e^{-\mu_B} + e^{-a\mu_B} - e^{-(a+1)\mu_B}$$

Although from the shape of a titration curve it should theoretically be possible to deduce the stoichiometry of cell interaction, we have to bear in mind that in most instances we cannot produce enough detailed and reliable data to make this kind of evaluation. This issue will be considered in some detail in Chapter 6 on clonal partition analysis.

In Figure 5.6 theoretical curves for several different T to B ratios are shown.

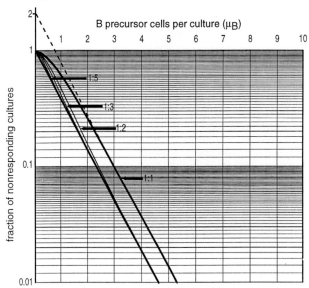

Figure 5.6. Two-target model. Different ratios of T and B cells. The curve labelled '1:1', when extrapolated to the *y* axis, intercepts it at value 2, as does the curve *m* = 2 of Figure 5.5

5.7 Levelling off

Let us consider a case where an experiment is designed to maintain 'saturating' levels of T cells, while titrating the B-cell input. Obviously, we would expect in such a case to observe single-hit kinetics. If we now perform the same analysis but with stepwise reductions in T-cell multiplicity we will eventually observe a levelling off phenomenon in the B-cell titration. Mathematically this would be explained by the following calculations.

Let us here use the same formula as we derived for the two-target events:

$$F_0 = 1 - \left(1 - e^{-\mu_B}\right)\left(1 - e^{-\mu_T}\right)$$

$$F_0 = e^{-\mu_B} + e^{-\mu_T} - e^{-(\mu_B + \mu_T)}$$

but instead of changing both μ_B and μ_T simultaneously (as was the case in the previous section) we keep μ_T constant.

For $\mu_T = 5$ and 2 and 1, we obtain the following formulae:

$$\mu_T = 5 \qquad F_0 = 0.007 + 0.99 e^{-\mu_B}$$

$$\mu_T = 2 \qquad F_0 = 0.135 + 0.86 e^{-\mu_B}$$

$$\mu_T = 1 \qquad F_0 = 0.37 \ + 0.63 e^{-\mu_B}$$

As can be seen from Figure 5.7, the constants 0.007, 0.135, 0.37, etc., are the asymptotes at which the titration curves level off.

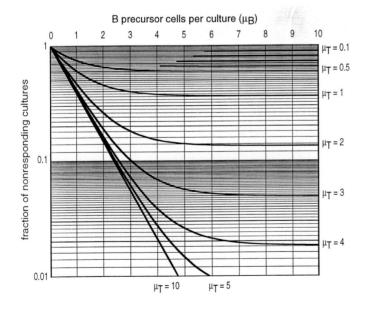

Figure 5.7.
Levelling off

5.8   Clone size

5.8.1   *Basic requirements*

The clonal selection theory (Jerne, 1955; Burnet, 1957) which has served as the theoretical framework of immunology over the past 40 years, postulates that precommitted cells interact with antigen and thereby are triggered to form a clone of antibody-forming cells. Obviously, *families of clones* are formed when an animal is stimulated with antigen, or when a culture containing several million lymphocytes is induced. Under limiting dilution conditions a certain fraction of cultures will contain *single clones*.

Although in most instances the term 'clone' implies the progeny of precursor cells which are capable of producing specific antibody, we have to remind ourselves of the following important feature of clonal proliferation. There are three processes occurring simultaneously during the evolution of a clone: *proliferation*, *maturation* and *death*. The bulk of a proliferating clone does not secrete antibody, while some members of the clone mature to become antibody-forming cells. These latter cells contribute very little to overall clonal proliferation. Thus, the clone itself has a *cryptic component* (vegetative pool) and a *productive component* (active clone).

The clone size estimation considered in this section is based upon the productive component – the active clone. Cells from a certain number of microcultures are assayed for the plaque-forming cell (PFC) content. The total number of PFC in the pool is designated as ΣPFC. The number of precursor cells (i.e. the number of induced clones) is calculated by separate means, as described earlier.

The average clone size $\bar{c}$, is then $\bar{c} = \dfrac{\Sigma\text{PFC}}{n}$

where n is the number of clones present in the pool used for the PFC assay.

5.9   Ratio of single clones over responding cultures

It is clear that when a low dose of cells is used as one of the points of the titration, the response in most of the wells originates from a single precursor cell. In Figure 5.8 the relevant curves are shown:

(i)   fraction of nonresponding cultures $\left(F_0 = e^{-\mu}\right)$

(ii)   fraction of singles $\left(F_1 = \mu e^{-\mu}\right)$

(iii)   ratio of cultures containing single clones over responding wells

$$\frac{S}{R} = \frac{F_1}{1 - F_0} = \frac{\mu \, e^{-\mu}}{1 - e^{-\mu}} = \frac{\mu \, e^{-\mu}}{1 - e^{-\mu}} \times \frac{e^{\mu}}{e^{\mu}} = \frac{\mu}{e^{\mu} - 1}$$

(iv)   fraction of impure cultures (doubles + triples + etc.)

$$F_{\text{impure}} = 1 - \left(F_0 + F_1\right) = 1 - \left(1 + \mu\right) e^{-\mu}$$

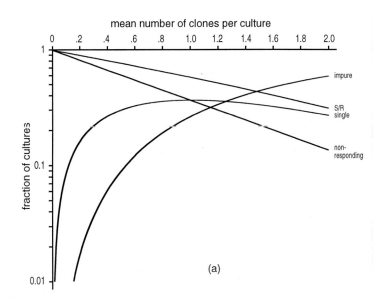

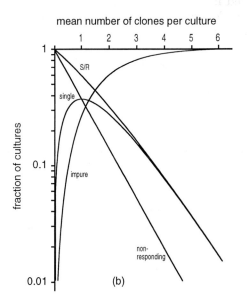

Figure 5.8. Single clones versus impure cultures. (a) Narrow range of μ (0 – 2); (b) complete relevant range of μ

5.10   Fraction of wells containing 0, 1, 2, 3 ... clones

With increasing μ, the fraction of wells containing r number of precursor cells increases up to a certain point, and when the 'overlap' becomes high the wells with r cells diminish. The maxima for the curves are calculated from the first derivation of the Poisson function.

$$F_r = \frac{\mu^r}{r!}e^{-\mu}$$

$$\frac{dF_r}{d\mu} = \frac{r\mu^{r-1}}{r!}e^{-\mu} - \frac{\mu^r}{r!}e^{-\mu}$$

$$\frac{dF_r}{d\mu} = 0$$

$$r\mu^{r-1} = \mu^r$$

$$r = \mu$$

This is to say that the maximum fraction of singles is obtained when the mean is one, and the maximum fraction of doubles is obtained when the mean is two, etc.

The value of F_r at the maxima is calculated by equating $\mu = r$ in the Poisson function.

$$F_r = \frac{r^r}{r!}e^{-r}$$

$$F_1 = e^{-1} = 0.37$$

$$F_2 = 2\,e^{-2} = 0.27$$

$$F_3 = 4.5\,e^{-3} = 0.225$$

$$F_4 = 10.7\,e^{-4} = 0.19$$

The relevant curves demonstrating this are shown in Figure 5.9.

Clone size. Clone size is defined as the number of progeny cells originating from a single precursor cell. In the case of antibody forming cells the clone size refers to the productive component of the clone, i.e. to the cells which actively secrete specific antibody.

Burst size. The progeny cells from several B precursor cells, induced by a single T cell, give the burst size.

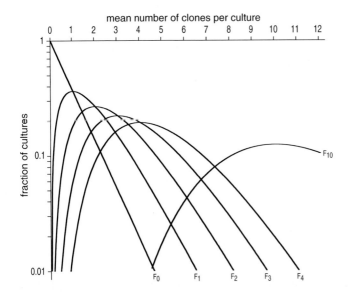

Figure 5.9. Fraction of wells containing 0, 1, 2, 3 ... clones

6   Models of clonal partition analysis

Let us imagine that we have a cell population which contains members that
need to cooperate to produce a response but also has members that are inhibitory to that response. If we were to take this large cell population and partition
it into small aliquots, then we might silence a cell which could have responded,
or alternatively derepress a cell which would have been unresponsive in the
larger population.

Partitioning in this way has often enabled the experimenter to observe
complex cellular interactions that might otherwise have remained unnoticed.
Graphical display of the responses often provided unusual titration curves
with V shapes; saw-tooth, zig-zag and other similar descriptions.

In earlier studies (Lefkovits and Waldmann, 1984; Waldmann and Lefkovits,
1984) we suggested that a formal distinction be made between the two applications: limiting dilution analysis (to obtain frequency estimation) and partition
analysis (to analyse cooperative responses). We will retain this distinction in
this monograph.

While most of the chapters of this volume can stand alone, this one is of
more value when considered in the context of the previous chapter. A multi-
target curve – described in section 5.6 – can be considered from two different
viewpoints. *First*, we might want to alter the experimental conditions by
admixing some cells, the limitation of which cause a 'targetness effect', and our
aim is to abrogate a targetness effect in order to obtain a single-hit shape which
safeguards the correct estimation of frequency. *Second*, we might want to study
the processes of cellular interactions, conditions for stimulatory/inhibitory
effects and the ratios in which the cells interact. The former consideration
defines the experiment as a 'limiting dilution analysis', the latter one as a 'partition analysis'.

6.1   Modelling the behaviour of cell populations that contain a
mixture of stimulatory and inhibitory cells

If we were to titrate a cell preparation containing suppressor cells into a population harbouring saturating numbers of target cells (be it B cells, T-helper cells
or any other cells) we would expect to obtain single-hit or multi-hit titration
curves. A single-hit curve would result if the presence of a single suppressor
cell in a culture is capable of preventing the response, while a multi-hit curve
would be obtained if more than one cell is needed to silence a culture. The

actual semi-log plot would be based on the 'fraction of responding cultures', since the *responding* cultures are those which *lack* the suppressor cell.

In this section we will address a more complex situation:

(i)   T-helper precursor cells and T-suppressor cells (or in more general terms 'stimulatory' and 'inhibitory' cells) are an integral part of the titrated cell population.

(ii) B-cell precursors, i.e. the responding cell population, are present in excess (saturating dose, or a multiplicity which for all practical purposes ensures the presence of at least one B cell/well).

We will consider two distinct cases which we call the 'dominance model' and the 'ratio dominance model'. The characteristics of these models are:

Dominance model	Ratio dominance model
B-precursor cells and accessory cells are supplied in saturating doses	B-precursor cells are supplied with a known multiplicity (known μ_B) which for all practical purposes fulfils the criteria for a saturating dose
T-helper precursors and T-suppressor cells are introduced only in the titrated samples	T-helper precursors and T-suppressor cells are introduced only in the titrated samples
A single suppressor cell, if present in a culture, will inactivate the whole culture	One suppressor cell is capable of silencing only a certain number of B-precursor cells

6.1.1   Dominance model

A single inhibitory cell, if present in a culture, will inactivate the whole culture.

Fraction of wells not containing suppressor cells $\quad e^{-\mu_{Ts}}$

Fraction of wells not containing helper cells $\quad e^{-\mu_{Th}}$

Fraction of wells not containing suppressor cells but containing at least one helper cell $\quad \left(1 - e^{-\mu_{Th}}\right)e^{-\mu_{Ts}}$

Fraction of nonresponding cultures

$$F_0 = 1 - \left(1 - e^{-\mu_{Th}}\right)e^{-\mu_{Ts}}$$

$$F_0 = 1 - e^{-\mu_{Ts}} + e^{-(\mu_{Th} + \mu_{Ts})}$$

T_h and T_s are introduced in the same sample, thus the ratio of the two kinds of cell is constant throughout the whole titration.

$$\frac{\mu_{Th}}{\mu_{Ts}} = R$$

$$F_0 = 1 - e^{-\mu_{Ts}} + e^{-(R+1)\mu_{Ts}}$$

or

$$F_0 = 1 - e^{-\frac{1}{R}\mu_{Th}} + e^{-\frac{R+1}{R}\mu_{Th}}$$

In Figures 6.1–6.3 curves of the combined helper and suppressor cell titration are shown with three different ratios of helper/suppressor cells. Both F_0
and F_+ curves are drawn. Note that the ratio of the slopes of the two curves (F_0
and F_+) is the chosen ratio of μ_{Th}/μ_{Ts}.

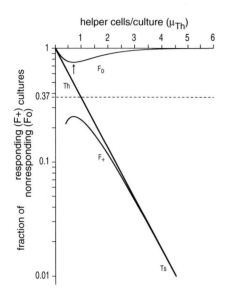

Figure 6.1. Titration of a mixture of T-helper and T-suppressor cells. Theoretical curves based on a dominance model for $R = 1$ (ratio helper/suppressor cells). Minimum $\mu_{Th} = 0.69$

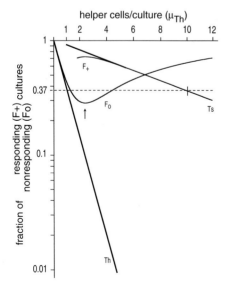

Figure 6.2. Titration of a mixture of T-helper and T-suppressor cells. Theoretical curves based on a dominance model for $R = 10$ (ratio helper/suppressor cells). Minimum $\mu_{Th} = 2.40$

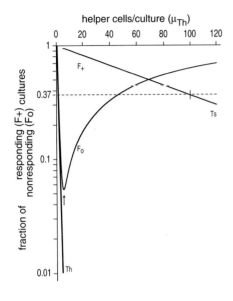

helper cells/culture (μ_{Th})

Figure 6.3. Titration of a mixture of T-helper and T-suppressor cells. Theoretical curves based on a dominance model for $R = 100$ (ratio helper/suppressor cells). Minimum $\mu_{Th} = 4.62$

We shall calculate the 'minima' of the titration curves from the zero term of the first derivation of the above function.

$$F_0 = 1 - e^{-\frac{1}{R}\mu_{Th}} + e^{-\frac{R+1}{R}\mu_{Th}}$$

$$\frac{dF_0}{d\mu_{Th}} = \frac{1}{R}e^{-\frac{1}{R}\mu_{Th}} - \frac{R+1}{R}e^{-\frac{R+1}{R}\mu_{Th}}$$

$$\frac{dF_0}{d\mu_{Th}} = 0 \text{ (for minima)}$$

It follows that:

$$\frac{1}{R}e^{-\frac{1}{R}\mu_{Th}} = \frac{R+1}{R}e^{-\frac{R+1}{R}\mu_{Th}}$$

$$e^{-\frac{1}{R}\mu_{Th}} = (R+1)e^{-\frac{R+1}{R}\mu_{Th}}$$

$$e^{-\frac{1}{R}\mu_{Th}} \times e^{\frac{R+1}{R}\mu_{Th}} = R+1$$

$$e^{\left(\frac{R+1}{R} - \frac{1}{R}\right)\mu_{Th}} = R+1$$

$$e^{\mu_{Th}} = R+1$$

$$\mu_{Th} = \ln(R+1)$$

Thus for the titration curves shown on Figures 6.1–6.3 the minima are

for R = 1 $\mu_{Th} = \ln 2 = 0.69$

for R = 10 $\mu_{Th} = \ln 11 = 2.40$

for R = 100 $\mu_{Th} = \ln 101 = 4.62$

which are also indicated by arrows on the corresponding figures.

6.1.2   Ratio–dominance model

One suppressor cell is capable of preventing the response of only a certain number of B-precursor cells.

Fraction of wells not containing suppressor cells	$e^{-\mu_{Ts}}$
Fraction of wells not containing helper cells	$e^{-\mu_{Th}}$
Multiplicity of B cells/culture	μ_B
Number of B cells inactivated by a single suppressor cell	n_B
Number of suppressor cells required to inactivate a culture	$a = \dfrac{\mu_B}{n_B}$

Sum of the fractions of cultures which will have less than a suppressor cells:

$$\left(1 + \mu_{Ts} + \frac{\mu_{Ts}^2}{2} + \ldots + \frac{\mu_{Ts}^{a-1}}{(a-1)!}\right) e^{-\mu_{Ts}}$$

Fraction of wells containing less than a suppressor cells but containing at least one helper cell

$$\left(1 + \mu_{Ts} + \frac{\mu_{Ts}^2}{2} + \ldots + \frac{\mu_{Ts}^{a-1}}{(a-1)!}\right)\left(1 - e^{-\mu_{Th}}\right) e^{-\mu_{Ts}}$$

$$F_0 = 1 - \left(1 + \mu_{Ts} + \frac{\mu_{Ts}^2}{2} + \ldots + \frac{\mu_{Ts}^{a-1}}{(a-1!)}\right)\left(1 - e^{-\mu_{Th}}\right) e^{-\mu_{Ts}}$$

Upon replacing $\mu_{Ts} = \dfrac{1}{R}\mu_{Th}$ (for the definition of R see p.95) we obtain

$$F_0 = 1 - \left(1 + \frac{1}{R}\mu_{Th} + \frac{1}{R^2} \times \frac{\mu_{Th}^2}{2} + \ldots + \frac{1}{R^{a-1}} \times \frac{\mu_{Th}^{a-1}}{(a-1)!}\right)\left(1 - e^{-\mu_{Th}}\right) e^{-\frac{1}{R}\mu_{Th}}$$

for R = 10, a = 3 $F_0 = 1 - \left(1 + \dfrac{1}{10}\mu_{Th} + \dfrac{1}{100} \times \dfrac{\mu_{Th}^2}{2}\right)\left(1 - e^{-\mu_{Th}}\right) e^{-\frac{1}{10}\mu_{Th}}$

for R = 10, a = 2 $F_0 = 1 - \left(1 + \dfrac{1}{10}\mu_{Th}\right)\left(1 - e^{-\mu_{Th}}\right) e^{-\frac{1}{10}\mu_{Th}}$

for R = 10, a = 1 $F_0 = 1 - \left(1 - e^{-\mu_{Th}}\right) e^{-\frac{1}{10}\mu_{Th}}$

In Figure 6.4 the curves for a ratio–dominance model for the fixed ratio of helper and suppressor cells, $R = 10$, and $a = 1, 2, 3$ are shown.

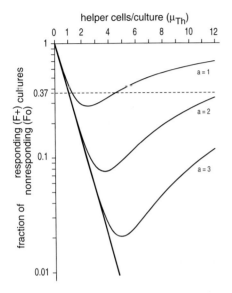

Figure 6.4. Titration of a mixture of T-helper and T-suppressor cells. Ratio-dominance model. *a*, number of suppressor cells required to activate a culture. *R*, ratio of helper/suppressor cells ($R = 10$)

The model we have provided deals with V-type curves. Sometimes the situation is more complex with so-called 'zig-zag' curves which most people have interpreted in a 3-cell model (i.e. a high frequency responding cell a lower frequency inhibitor, and a lower frequency responder that is not inhibited). Dozmorov and coworkers (1995a, b, 1996) have devised a model to explain these zig-zag patterns employing a simple 2-cell model for which they have tested favourably against their own experimental data, as shown next.

6.2 Dozmorov model

Although saw-tooth and zig-zag curves have been reported in many previous experimental studies, no one has analysed their data as thoroughly as Dozmorov *et al.* (1995a, 1996), culminating in the development of a new two-cell model and a range of mathematical formulae with which we can systematically analyse such curves.

6.2.1 Regulatory interactions between virgin and memory T cells

Dozmorov and Miller (1996) have shown that LDA of virgin CD4 T cells yields single-hit kinetics, that LDA of memory CD4 T cells results in a multi-hit form of the curve and, moreover, that the mixture of both gave a zig-zag curve.

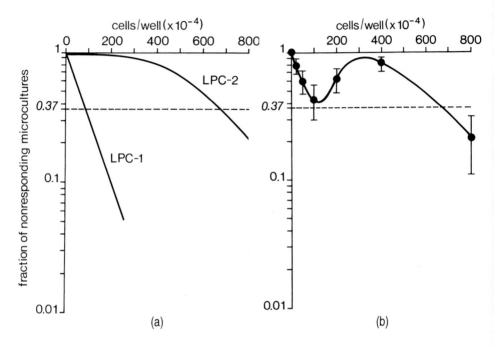

Figure 6.5. Illustration of the two-cell model for interactions between virgin and memory T cells in limiting dilution cultures. (a) Theoretical curves for LPC-1 and LPC-2, (b) experimental curve for the mixture of LPC-1 and LPC-2

The addition of IL-10, anti-IL-10 antibody or IL-2 converts or blocks some of the events, details of which are given in the above reference.

6.2.2 Dozmorov's nonlinear two-cell model

Dozmorov scrutinised LDA curves of the type 'response–inhibition–response' and suggested that the three components of the response can be accommodated in a two-cell model. The basis of the model is as follows.

Two cell types, LPC-1 and LPC-2, are involved in the response (Figure 6.5).

(i)   LPC-1 produces a single-hit kinetic response.

(ii) LPC-2 is capable of suppressing a response or it produces a response on its own depending on the number of cells. The LPC-2 population exerts its activity in a multi-hit fashion.

(iii) When the culture contains m or more cells (LPC-2), an inhibitory effect results.

(iv) When the culture contains n or more cells (LPC-2), a positive response is generated.

(v) n is always a larger number than m.

Their formulae, based on the above assumptions, require the use of iterative algorithms, the implementation of which is not a straightforward issue. With a few simplifying assumptions a set of equations was derived which gave satisfactory estimates of the model parameters. The Dozmorov procedure is shown in the following example (modified from Dozmorov *et al.*, 1996) in a step by step fashion.

(i) We estimate the cell dose containing a single LPC-1 (from a single-hit model) (Figure 6.6).

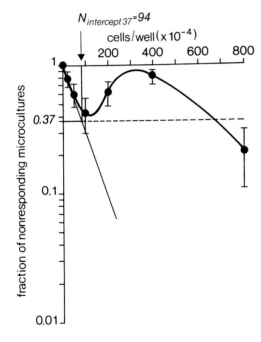

$$N_{\text{intercept } 37\%} = 94 \text{ cells}$$

$$f_1 = \frac{1}{94} = 0.0106$$

Figure 6.6. Estimation of the frequency of LPC-1 cells

(ii) We estimate the cell dose containing a single LPC-2 (from a multi-hit model) (Figure 6.7).

The aim of *limiting dilution analysis* is to obtain frequency estimates. The aim of *partition analysis* is to investigate cooperative responses. Partition analysis does not lead to acceptance or rejection of a null hypothesis, though it provides models for the adequate interpretation of complex titration curves.

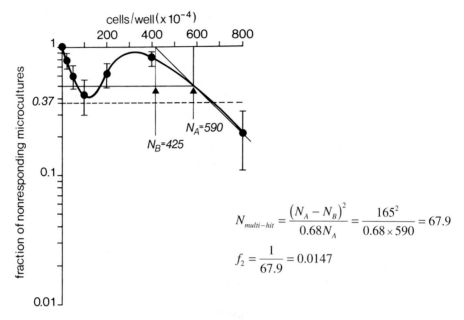

Figure 6.7. Estimation of the frequency of LPC-2 cells

(iii) We estimate the parameter m, with the property that cultures having m cells (or more) will score negative (Figure 6.8):

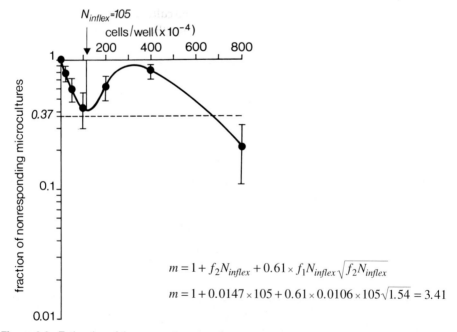

Figure 6.8. Estimation of the parameters m and n

(iv)   We estimate the parameter n with the property that cultures having n cells (or more) will score positive (Figure 6.8).

$$n = 1 + f_2 N_A$$
$$n = 1 + 0.0147 \times 590 = 9.67$$

Summary. The cell population contains LPC-1 at a frequency 0.0106 (1/94) and LPC 2 at a frequency 0.0147 (1/67.9).

- Cultures containing LPC-1 and missing LPC-2 will respond.
- Cultures containing one to three LPC-2 fail to interfere with the response.
- Cultures containing LPC-1 and four to nine LPC-2 will suppress the response.
- Cultures containing 10 or more LPC-2 score as responding.

The curve minimum is achieved when the input of cells is such that any further cell dose increase yields more suppressed cultures (i.e. those containing four to nine LPC-2), than additionally induced productive cultures (i.e. those which gain an LPC-1). The curve maximum is achieved when the input of cells is such that any further cell dose increase diminishes the portion of cultures containing four to nine LPC-2. The beginning of the suppression may be determined as cell input, when at least one culture with one LPC-1 will contain four LPC-2. The beginning of the LPC-2 own activity will be seen when there appears at least one culture with 10 LPC-2. We shall exemplify these conditions for an instance of 120 cultures. We shall ask the following two questions:

(i)   At what cell dose do we expect at least one culture containing one LPC-1 and four LPC-2?

(ii)   At what cell dose do we expect at least one culture with 10 LPC-2?

The answer to these questions is given by solving the following two equations:

(i)
$$\left(1 - e^{-f_1 T}\right) \times e^{-f_2 T} \times e \frac{(f_2 T)^4}{4!} \times 120 = 1$$

for $f_1 = 1/94$, $f_2 = 1/68$ the solution is: T = 70 cells / well

(ii)
$$e^{-f_2 T} \times \frac{(f_2 T)^{10}}{4!} \times 120 = 1$$

for $f_2 = 1/68$ the solution is: T = 290 cells / well

If the reader does not wish to make the effort which is required to solve the above equations, he/she can check the validity of the analysis by substituting

in the first equation for $f_1 = 1/94$, $f_2 = 1/68$ and T=70, and

in the second one for $f_1 = 1/94$, $f_2 = 1/68$ and T=290.

Thus, at a cell input of 70 cells/well, one culture (out of 120) has suppressive conditions, and at a cell input of 290 cells there is one culture (out of 120) with the property of overcoming the suppression.

Note that when less replicate cultures are considered (i.e. 24 instead of 120), the cell dose at which the cultures of type (i) and (ii) appear is higher (T = 110 and T = 410). The curve minimum and maximum is not altered.

7 Exemplary experimental systems and titration protocols

7.1 Media, antigens, mitogens and cells

So many workers have improvised and evolved new protocols to exploit LDA in mouse and man that it would be inappropriate for us to select just a few for this monograph. Rather, we would prefer to invite workers in the field to contribute their own protocols to a website which will be initiated on publication of this book. For those who would like to 'practise' some of the principles in the well-tested murine models of T–B cooperation we provide below a minimal starter kit.

7.1.1 Preparation of cell suspensions

Most of the experiments to be discussed in this monograph have been performed with mouse spleen cells.

Spleen cells

Mice are killed by cervical dislocation. Their spleens are removed aseptically and placed into sterile Petri dishes containing appropriately buffered chilled balanced salt solution (BSS). The cells are gently teased, using a pair of surgical forceps. The suspension is then transferred into a sterile plastic tube and kept for 2-3 min on ice to allow clumps to settle. The suspension is transferred – without the clumps – into a sterile plastic centrifuge tube and the cells are centrifuged in a cooled centrifuge at 200 x g for 10 min. The cells are resuspended in a small volume of culture medium, counted and brought to a required final cell density.

Formula: *modified Mishell–Dutton* (Mishell and Dutton, 1967)

  100   ml MEM for suspension cultures
     1   ml L-glutamine (200 mM)
     1   ml nonessential amino acids (100x)
     1   ml sodium pyruvate (100 mM)
     1   ml streptomycin and penicillin mixture (5000 U/ml each)
     2   ml HEPES (1 M)
  0.3 ml 2-mercaptoethanol (14 mM)
  5.5 ml foetal calf serum

Formula: *Schreier* (Schreier and Nordin, 1977)

   80   ml RPMI 1640
     1   ml L-glutamine (200 mM)
     1   ml streptomycin and penicillin mixture (5000 U/ml each)
  0.3 ml 2-mercaptoethanol (14 mM)
   20   ml foetal calf serum (heat inactivated)

Antigens

Sheep erythrocytes (SRBC), donkey erythrocytes (DRBC) and horse erythrocytes (HRBC) are used from individual, tested donors. Red cells are stored in Alsever's solution.

Keyhole limpet haemocyanin (KLH) can be obtained from Calbiochem. Fowl IgG (FGG) is prepared by multiple ammonium sulphate precipitation according to the procedure described by Miller and Warner (1971). Ovalbumin (OA) is obtained from Sigma Chemical Company, St. Louis, MO. Trinitrophenylated proteins TNP-KLH, TNP-FGG, TNP-OA are prepared by a modified Rittenberg and Amkraut method (1966).

7.1.2 Abrogation of B-cell activity

Precursor B-cell function can be abrogated by treatment with Mitomycin C. To achieve this 2×10^7-4×10^7 spleen cells are incubated with 40 µg/ml Mitomycin C for 20 min in BSS. After this, the cells are washed and then centrifuged through a layer of foetal calf serum in order to remove residual Mitomycin C.

Precursor B-cell function can also be eliminated by irradiation with a dose of 1200 rads. Irradiated nude spleen cells are conveniently used as filler cells.

7.1.3 Depletion of T cells

(i) Anti-Thy 1 treatment

Monoclonal antibodies against the Thy 1 antigen are now commercially available. The dilutions of reagents used do of course depend upon the relative activities of preparations and should always be determined in functional tests. We have found it advisable to routinely absorb guinea pig complement or rabbit complement with mouse spleen cells prior to use. 'Batch-killing' of T cells is performed by two-stage manoeuvres. Firstly, cells are preincubated at 0°C with the anti-Thy 1 reagent for 30 min (appropriately diluted), and then the cells are washed once and incubated with complement (i.e. serum) for a further 30 min at 37°C, washed again and then collected after spinning through foetal calf serum.

(ii) ATxBM mice

Thymectomy of young adult mice is performed by the method of Miller (1960). Approximately 4 weeks after thymectomy, mice are irradiated with 875 rads and injected intravenously with about 4×10^6 syngeneic bone marrow cells. The spleens of thymectomized and bone marrow-reconstituted mice (ATxBM) are used 5-12 weeks later, as a source of B cells.

7.1.4   Depletion of B cells. Enrichment of T cells

The most convenient method to deplete cell populations of B cells is the nylon wool column method described by Julius *et al.*, (1973). 0.6 g purified nylon wool is packed into the barrel of 12 ml plastic syringes, autoclaved, rinsed with Dulbecco's PBS, and drained of excess medium.

A total of $1-1.5 \times 10^8$ cells in a volume of 2 ml BSS is loaded onto the column, and incubated for 45 min at 37°C, and then the cells are eluted with BSS. The effluent lymphoid population contains close to 90% T cells and less than 5% B cells.

However, red cells are also not retained on the columns and therefore the effluent cell population has a greater proportion of red cells, compared to the starting material. One way of removing red cells is to use the ammonium chloride method whereby the nylon wool passed T cells are incubated in 2 ml of Gey's BSS (where the sodium chloride is wholly replaced by ammonium chloride). After 10 min at 0°C, a great excess of BSS is added to the tube and the ammonium chloride removed by washing and spinning through foetal calf serum. Most red cells are lost by this manoeuvre while the T-cell function remains intact.

7.1.5   Preparation of cell mixtures

There are two important points to keep in mind for this section:

(i)   one has to work within a relatively narrow range of cell densities for optimal culture conditions; thus, if very dilute populations of cells have to be used, then some source of filler cells (see section 5.2) often has to be employed;

(ii)   it is necessary to ensure that all cell populations (except the one which is titrated, see sections 5.2 and 5.4) are well represented, or in other words, are saturating. The sorts of cell mixtures adopted have usually contained nonirradiated B cells, irradiated B cells, nonirradiated or irradiated T cells, and macrophages.

In the previous section it was pointed out that if we use the term B-cell populations, we mean nude spleen cells or anti-Thy 1 and complement-treated normal spleen cells or cells from ATxBM mice (see section 7.1.3). If we use the term T-cell populations, it might mean nylon purified T cells, 'educated' T cells or, sometimes, normal spleen cells when the B-cell activity can be disregarded. The terms active and inactive B cells are reserved for nonirradiated and irradiated B cells, respectively.

The mixing protocol changes from experiment to experiment depending on the nature of the problem to be studied. For illustration we describe here two typical protocols, one for a B-cell titration, and one for a T-cell titration.

Mixing protocol for B-cell titration

Spleen cells from nude mice are the source of B cells. They are titrated over the range 0-2 x 10^5 active nude cells per microculture. A functional excess of T-helper activity is ensured by complementation with, for example, splenic T cells from mice previously immunised to SRBC. The number of T cells added is kept constant at say, 5 x 10^4 per microculture. Any contribution of contaminating B cells to the response is prevented by irradiation of the T cells (see section 7.1.2). Constant cell density is maintained by compensating the titrated active nude spleen cells with irradiated nude spleen cells. Since the function of macrophages in this system is thought to be radioresistant, the constant cell density ensures a constant supply of macrophage activity.

Table 7.1. B-cell titration protocol

	Irradiated T cells	Irradiated nude cells	Active nude cells	SRBC 50 µl of 1%	Active nude cells per 10 µl culture
a	0.5 ml	1.5 ml	–	+	0
b	0.5 ml	1.0 ml	0.5 ml	+	5 x 10^4
c	0.5 ml	0.5 ml	1 ml	+	1 x 10^5
d	0.5 ml	–	1.5 ml	+	1.5 x 10^5
e	–	–	2 ml	+	2 x 10^5

Cell density for all three stock cell suspensions is 2 x 10^7/ml. Final cell density for all five groups is 2 x 10^7/ml. Group *a* negative control; group *e* response without added T cell activity.

Mixing protocol for T-cell titration

The principle is the same as for B-cell titration. However, in this case each microculture well contains one or more B-precursor cells, whilst the T cells are limiting.

The cell density of the stock nude spleen cell suspension is 3.0 x 10^7/ml. The cell density of the stock T-cell suspension is 2 x 10^7/ml. The final cell density is therefore not constant (range 1.5 x 10^7-2.1 x 10^7). Irradiated T cells cannot be

Table 7.2. T-cell titration protocol

	Active nude cells	Medium	Helper T cells	SRBC 50 µl of 1%	Helper T cells per 10 µl culture
a	1 ml	1 ml	–	+	0
b	1 ml	0.8 ml	0.2 ml	+	2×10^4
c	1 ml	0.6 ml	0.4 ml	+	4×10^4
d	1 ml	0.4 ml	0.6 ml	+	6×10^4

used as fillers for keeping the cell density constant, because irradiation does not necessarily abolish the helper activity of helper cells and irradiated cells would thus contribute to the response. Fillers have not proven essential in experiments examining helper function.

The experimenter is expected to establish in preliminary experiments the 'adequate' dose of B cells. With a mean of three B-precursor cells per well 5% of wells are expected to contain no B-precursor cells. It is recommended to work with at least five B-precursor cells per well to ensure saturation.

Note: Both protocols are only examples; unlimited numbers of variations may be introduced. The most common variation is the source of B and T cells, or, alternatively, the use of available helper factors derived from T cells instead of saturating numbers of T cells. The source of filler cells may also vary (e.g. irradiated thymocytes or irradiated spleen cells from B mice, or irradiated cell lines).

7.1.6   The dispensing of cells into microculture trays

Once the cell mixture is prepared and antigen added, the cell suspension is drawn into a multi-syringe dispenser. Then 10 µl are dispensed into each of the sixty wells of a tissue culture tray (Falcon Microtest 3034); about 0.4 ml of medium is pipetted into the peripheral groove, in order to maintain the humidity, and then the plates are covered. The trays are then incubated at 37°C in a humid sealed container in an atmosphere of 83% of N_2, 10% CO_2, and 7% O_2.

7.1.7   Maintenance of microcultures

A standard experiment takes 3-7 days. If the microcultures are performed in MEM, daily feeding with maintenance medium (nutritional cocktail) is necessary. Cultures performed in RPMI medium (formula Schreier) do not need to be fed.

Feeding can be efficiently performed by the use of a sterile multi-syringe dispenser, 1 µl of the maintenance medium is added to each well by lowering the droplets onto the surface of the microculture. The incubation box is re-gassed after feeding and further incubated at 37°C. Frequent opening of the sealed container is to be avoided, as some of the medium in the wells will evaporate.

Formula: maintenance medium (nutritional feeding cocktail)

15	ml Eagle's MEM
2	ml essential amino acids (50x)
1	ml nonessential amino acids (100x)
1	ml L-glutamine (200 mM)
3	ml sodium bicarbonate (7.5%)
0.4	ml glucose (50%)
10	ml foetal calf serum

7.1.8   *Priming schedules for obtaining optimal T and B-memory cells*

Mice are primed i.p. with 200-500 µg KLH in Freund's complete adjuvant, followed 4 weeks later by 50-100 µg KLH i.p. (without adjuvant). After 1-5 weeks, the spleens of these mice provide a good source of T-helper cells specific for KLH. Repeated booster doses 1 week prior to harvest provide reliable helper activity.

Spleen cells from mice primed previously with 200-500 µg TNP-OA or TNP-FGG in Freund's complete adjuvant followed by soluble boosters are used as a source of hapten-primed B cells. If cells are taken 7-14 days after boosting then they are a rich source of IgG memory cells.

SRBC-educated thymus cells or KLH-educated thymus cells are obtained by injecting 10^8 thymocytes and 0.1 ml of 10% SRBC or KLH with or without adjuvant into 875 rads irradiated mice. Spleen cells from such mice are the source of educated T cells.

Anti-SRBC T-cell memory is induced by suboptimal doses of SRBC: 1×10^5-5×10^5 SRBC injected i.v. elicit no detectable antibody production, but 3-7 days or 14-21 days later the spleen cells are capable of supplying optimal helper activity. Larger doses of SRBC, e.g. 2×10^7, can be used to prime similarly for helper activity but the cells must be passed through nylon wool and treated with Mitomycin C to ensure optimal assessment of T-cell function.

7.2   Determination of the response

The reader will be aware of the range of methods for assessing antibody responses. In our first edition we described haemolytic assays in gel, plaque-forming cells, isoelectric focusing, radioimmunoassays and a range of other technologies. Since that time enzyme-linked immunosorbent assays have become commonplace, and would be for most purposes the most convenient. As there are now many technical manuals that give detailed protocols for measuring responses, and many devices for sampling from microtitre and microtest plates, there is no need for us to describe these in this volume. The reader is encouraged to select the assay most convenient for their circumstances. Some up-to-date protocols will be made available on the website. Since many experiments described in this monograph are based on the so-called 'spot test' a brief description follows.

7.2.1   *Spot test*

Samples of microcultures are aspirated with the replicator (Lefkovits, 1972; Lefkovits and Kamber, 1972) and released onto the assay plate. The assay plate is a 100 x 15 mm Petri dish with 1.4% agar bottom layer and 0.7% agarose top layer containing red cells. When the released droplets have soaked in, complement is added and the plates are incubated for 45 min at 37°. Zones of lysis mark the cultures which have produced antibody.

7.3   Titration of B-precursor cells

Here we are concerned with two aspects of limiting dilution analysis as applied to the immune system: (i) the experimental design, and (ii) the way data may be plotted graphically and subsequently analysed.

7.3.1   *Design*

First one has to establish what range of cell input needs to be tested. In preliminary experiments it is desirable to cover several orders of magnitude, while for the final test one can apply a linear selection from the 'useful range' (see also section 5.2).

Example:

Preliminary test:	10^3, 3×10^3, 10^4, 3×10^4, 10^5 cells/well
	result: 3×10^4 and higher input yielded all cultures positive.
Final test:	1×10^4, 2×10^4, 3×10^4 cells/well, or
	1×10^4, 1.5×10^4, 2×10^4, 2.5×10^4, 3×10^4 cells/well.

Second, one needs to decide on the number of cultures to be analysed. The rule of thumb is not to use less than 60 cultures per experimental point. The reason for this is clarified in section 4.6 on confidence limits.

Third, it is important to choose a neutral source of filler cells. Irradiated B cells (irradiated nude spleen cells or irradiated anti-Thy 1-treated spleen cells) are the most convenient. If other types of filler cells are to be used, one must ensure that these in no way disturb or contribute to the response analysed. In general, irradiation of filler cells is worthwhile, whatever the source.

Fourth, an excess of all other necessary components, like macrophages, T cells (in the case of T-dependent responses) or T-cell factors, has to be ensured.

In establishing these criteria, one should not rely on the information obtained from large cultures (macrocultures), and the relevant parameters should be established anew for the microcultures.

7.3.2   Plot

The results are plotted on semi-log graph paper; the fraction of nonresponding cultures (y axis) on a log scale, and the cell input (x axis) on a linear scale. For each experimental point the 95% confidence limits are read from a table (see section 4.6 and Appendix/3).

Table 7.3. Example (i)

		Number of responding cultures out of 60	Fraction of negative cultures F_0
Raw data:	no B cells	0	1
	5×10^4	40	0.33
	1×10^5	60	0
	1.5×10^5	60	0

Decision: an inadequate range was used; there is only one 'useful point'; therefore there is no sense in plotting these results

The results of example (i) are not plotted because there is only one 'useful' point, and so such results cannot be used as a serious basis for constructing a titration curve. They serve, however, as groundwork for planning a repeat experiment.

Table 7.4. Example (ii)

		Number of responding cultures out of 60	Fraction of negative cultures F_0
Raw data:	no B cells	0	1
	2×10^4	34	0.43
	4×10^4	51	0.15
	6×10^4	57	0.05
	1×10^5	60	0
	1.5×10^5	60	0

Decision: all data except those for the highest cell input (1.5×10^5) are plotted. The $F_0 = 0$ for 1×10^5 cell input is indicated by an arrow (see Figure 7.1)

Example (ii) is a successful experiment giving a straight line (Figure 7.1). At the intercept of the titration curve with the 37% F_0 line we read the corresponding sample size. In this example it is 21 000 cells. In other words, in a sample of 21 000 cells we can expect on average one precursor cell.

$$N = 21\,000$$

$$\text{frequency} = \frac{1}{N} = \frac{1}{21000} = 4.8 \times 10^{-5}$$

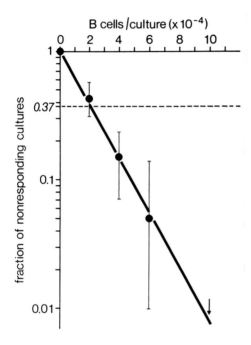

Figure 7.1. B-cell titration. Single-hit curve.
Frequency 4.8×10^{-5} (Data in Table 7.4)

Table 7.5. Example (iii)

		Number of responding cultures out of 60	Fraction of negative cultures F_0
Raw data:	no B cells	0	1
	2×10^4	2	0.97
	4×10^4	1	0.98
	6×10^4	11	0.82
	1×10^5	60	0
	1.5×10^5	60	0

Decision: all data except those for the highest cell input (1.5×10^5) are plotted. The $F_0 = 0$ for 1×10^5 cell input is indicated by an arrow (see Figure 7.2)

Example (iii) yields a curve (Figure 7.2) which would seem to be 'multi-hit'. However, the curve might easily be a multi-target curve, a multi-hit curve or a compound multi-target/multi-hit curve, but for convenience we call them all multi-hit curves (unless we are certain that we are dealing with multi-target curves). The golden rule at the present stage of the game is not to estimate the frequencies from such types of curve.

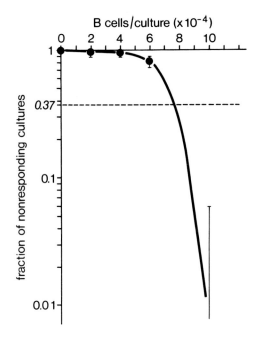

Figure 7.2. B-cell titration. Multi-hit curve. No frequency estimate. (Data in Table 7.5)

Table 7.6. Example (iv)

		Number of responding cultures out of 60	Fraction of negative cultures F_0
Raw data:	no B cells	0	1
	2×10^4	46	0.23
	4×10^4	53	0.12
	6×10^4	54	0.10
	1×10^5	52	0.13
	1.5×10^5	54	0.10

Decision: all data points are plotted (see Figure 7.3)

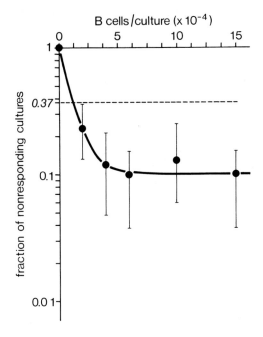

Figure 7.3. B-cell titration. Levelling-off curve.
Frequency 6.7 x 10⁻⁵. (Data in Table 7.6)

Example (iv) yields a curve (Figure 7.3) which demonstrates the phenomenon of 'levelling off'. Here the frequency can be estimated, since the intercept of the titration curve with the 37% line is within the linear portion:

$$N = 15\,000$$

$$\text{frequency} = \frac{1}{N} = \frac{1}{15\,000} = 6.7 \times 10^{-5}$$

The most reasonable explanation for 'levelling off' is that the 'multiplicity' of the T cells was too low, and a certain fraction of wells therefore did not receive any helper cells. This fraction of wells remained negative irrespective of the input of the titrated B-cell population.

7.4   Titration of T-helper cells

At first glance one might be tempted to say that there is nothing special to be learned about T-cell titrations that we have not already established from B-cell titrations. This is not entirely correct. We have to be aware of two crucial points:

(i)   although the titrated cell is a T cell, the functional assay is usually based on a B-cell response; and

(ii)   all cultures contain B cells in excess, and in many instances a considerable fraction of microcultures may respond without any external T-cell influence. In other words, our data analysis would be contaminated by a background effect.

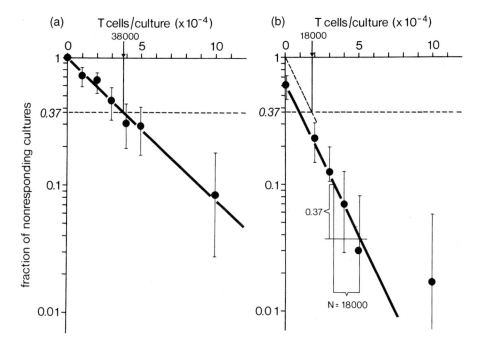

Figure 7.4. T-cell titration. (a) Single-hit curve. Frequency 2.6 x 10⁻⁵. (b) Single-hit curve; correction for background. Frequency 5.6 x 10⁻⁵

In Figure 7.4 the results of a standard T-cell titration experiment are plotted. In Figure 7.4a the titration curve is of a quality similar to that obtained for the B-cell titration in Figure 7.1 (previous section). Using the same procedure for frequency estimation we find:

$$N = 38\,000$$

$$\text{frequency} = \frac{1}{N} = \frac{1}{38\,000} = 2.6 \times 10^{-5}$$

In Figure 7.4b we see a titration curve from an experiment with a high background (a spontaneous response from the B cells alone) probably due to some residual contaminating T cells. To make a correct frequency estimate the curve must either be corrected for the background (by drawing a parallel straight line through the origin) and the frequency read from this corrected curve, or $\Delta F_0 = 0.37$ determined for that curve and ΔN cells read directly from it (Figure 5.4b). Both procedures yield:

$N = 18\,000$

$$\text{frequency} = \frac{1}{N} = \frac{1}{18\,000} = 5.6 \times 10^{-5}$$

7.5 Titration of a mixture of T-helper and T-suppressor cells

In Chapters 5 and 6 we tried to separate conceptually limiting dilution analysis from partition analysis. The analysis of a cell population containing T-helper cells and T-suppressor cells falls into the category of 'partition analysis'. But this does not need to be the case if our sole intention is to estimate the frequencies of Th or Ts cells.

We will examine the results of an experiment in which the analysed cell population contains MLR-enriched allogeneic T cells in combination with a 'saturating dose' of nude spleen cells and antigen (SRBC) (Corley *et al.*, 1978). The 'V shaped' titration curve shown in Figure 7.5 reveals that two cell populations – helper and suppressor – are present in the allogeneic mixture.

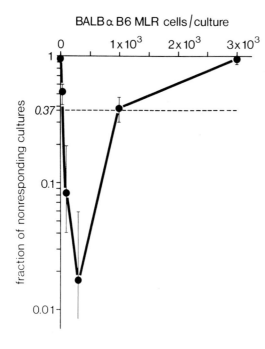

Figure 7.5. Titration of a mixture of T-helper and T-suppressor cells. MLR-enriched allogeneic T cells titrated into nude spleen cells; anti-SRBC response assayed by spot test

The slope of the portion of the curve indicating help is very steep. It is apparent that the intercept with the 37% line is in a range of less than 100 cells. In instances like this, one should redraw the data choosing an adequate scale. A separate plot for suppressor cells (using fractions of responding cultures) should be drawn as well. Figure 7.6 displays these plots.

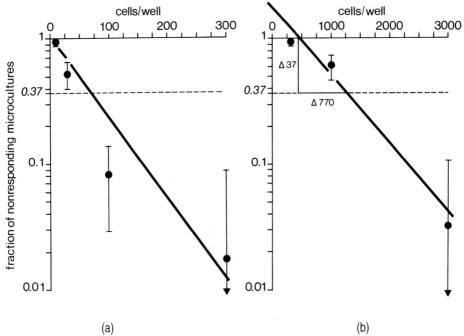

Figure 7.6. Plots of the helper portion (a) and the suppressor portion (b) of the MLR-enriched allogeneic cells titrated into nude spleen cells. The curves (a) and (b) represent the same data as given in Figure 7.5

In Figure 7.6a the 37% intercept corresponds to 70 cells

$$N_{Th} = 70 \text{ cells}$$

$$f = \frac{1}{70} = 0.0143$$

In Figure 7.6b the $\Delta 37\%$ corresponds to 700 cells

$$N_{Th} = 770 \text{ cells}$$

$$f = \frac{1}{770} = 1.3 \times 10^{-3}$$

Note that in Figure 7.6a the plot is based on F_0, while in Figure 7.6b it is based on F_+. The reason for this is explained in Chapters 3 and 4.

The plot in Figure 7.6b is based on a regression line disregarding the origin. Such a plot is usual when two competing populations are titrated.

It is known that allogeneic reactions can both enhance and suppress antibody responses. The interesting feature of such titration curves is that at a low input of the titrated cells the 'helper portion' is revealed, while at a higher input the suppressor activity dominates. When cultures of a larger size are used, this helper effect at low doses of allogeneic cells may be totally undetectable while intermediate and high doses of allogeneic cells suppress the response.

7.6   Titration of factor-producing cells

Much information exists about the interaction of T-helper factors with B-cell populations. Most of the data have been obtained from factors produced in bulk cultures of lymphocytes, but several attempts have been made to study these factors under limiting dilution conditions. The studies focused on T cells making non-specific helper factors (cytokines in the modern nomenclature).

Principle

A two-stage culture system was used, whereby in the first stage factor-containing supernatants are obtained from single helper T cells (achieved by limiting dilution), and in the second stage the supernatants are tested on samples of antigen-specific B cells.

Design

In *master cultures*, restricted numbers of cells are used to ensure single cell products in some of the cultures and to enable a full titration.
Convenient cell input:

3×10^3 cells/well

1×10^4 "   "

3×10^4 "   "

1×10^5 "   "

In *recipient cultures* a high multiplicity of B cells is used to ensure the presence of specific B-cell precursors in each culture.
Convenient cell input:

1×10^5 or 1.5×10^5 nude spleen cells/well.

Key features

In the first stage, the supernatants rather than the cells are transferred, thus potential allogeneic cell reactions are excluded in those experiments where co-operation across the H-2 barrier is studied. Furthermore, one can screen several samples from the product of a single factor-producing cell. For example, several aliquots from a single supernatant sample may be tested on replica recipient cultures for their capacity to help responses against a variety of antigens. This approach has been adopted in an attempt to examine B and T-cell subsets in the mouse; details of this approach will be elaborated in Chapter 8.

7.7   Clone size estimations

Clone size is the number of antibody-forming cells originating from a single B-precursor cell.

Burst size is a misnomer identifying the number of antibody-forming cells obtained from a certain (usually known) number of precursor cells. The number of PFC per culture well, in a B-cell titration, indicates the *clone size*, and in a T-cell titration it refers to the *burst size*.

Example 1:

60 microcultures were pooled and assayed for PFC; 2460 PFC were detected. By spot test, 27 cultures were identified as positive

$$F_0 = \frac{33}{60} = 0.55$$

$$\mu = -\ln F_0 = -\ln 0.55 = 0.6$$

$$n_{clones} = \mu \times w_T = 0.6 \times 60 = 36 \text{ clones}$$

$\left(w_T, \text{ total number of assayed microculture wells}\right)$

$$\Sigma PFC = 2460$$

$$\bar{c} = \frac{\Sigma PFC}{n} = \frac{2460}{36} = 68 \text{ PFC}$$

Example 2:

Individual microcultures are assayed for PFC content. The fraction of nonresponding cultures is calculated either on the basis of cultures in which no PFC were found,[*] or by performing an independent spot test, usually from another set of microcultures. Then the sum of the PFC is calculated (ΣPFC), and the clone size estimated, as shown above. Note that the values of PFC from individual wells are of no consequence for clone size calculations, and only the ΣPFC is used.

---

[*] We have made an arbitrary decision to consider as negative cultures those which contain zero PFC but also microcultures which contain 1 PFC. This may sometimes be erroneous, but we argue that 1 PFC might be a background PFC, or a non-dividing recruited cell not participating in clonal proliferation, or some other artifact.

Table 7.7. Example

	7	43		15	2
83	22				
	57	50			1
3	4	17	14	80	48
33	4	4			
				22	
		12	46	24	28
	43		42	14	1
18		18	2	76	15
		18	2		43

$\Sigma\text{PFC} = 909$ (disregarding 2 wells with 1 PFC)

w_R $= 33$ (w_R responding wells)

w_T $= 60$ (w_T, total wells analysed)

$$F_0 = \frac{27}{60} = 0.45$$

$$\mu = -\ln F_0 = -\ln 0.45 = 0.8$$

$$n_{\text{clones}} = \mu \times w_T = 0.8 \times 60 = 48 \text{ clones}$$

$$\bar{c} = \frac{\Sigma\text{PFC}}{n} = \frac{909}{48} = 18.7 \text{ PFC}$$

Example 3:

Cells are harvested from a conventional 1 ml culture and PFC content is assayed. The number of precursor cells is estimated from microcultures. The clone size calculation is performed as above. We do not recommend this method, because the efficiency of activation and clone size expansion might be different in the two systems. Note that the actual calculation would be the same as shown in examples 1 and 2.

7.8   Cumulative plot for clone sizes

We pointed out in the previous section that the values of PFC from individual wells are superfluous for estimating the clone size. The only PFC information required is the sum of PFC present in w_T total analysed microculture wells. The assay of individual wells does, however, supply important information on other aspects:

    (i)   it shows whether or not the sum of PFC is strongly influenced by extreme values,

(ii) it gives the experimenter a sense of whether or not all wells of the culture tray are experiencing equivalent/homogeneous culture conditions on the basis that one searches for monotonous progression of the ranked data rather than bi- or multimodal behaviour and

(iii) the resulting cumulative plot provides the reader with information on all the assay data of an experiment.

This information can be ascertained by using 'grouped plots' or 'cumulative plots' (Lefkovits *et al.*, 1975). In the 'grouped plot' we group wells containing 2-3 PFC, 4-7 PFC, 8-15 PFC, 16-31 PFC, etc., and present the data as a bar diagram (Figure 7.7). A criticism of this type of presentation is that the grouping itself implies a certain interpretation which we would not like to evoke. (It looks as if we are implying that each group reflects one cell division.) In the 'cumulative plot' we rank all values and plot each value. The cumulative plot is composed of two parts (Figure 7.8). The lower zone indicates the fraction of nonresponding cultures (F_0) and the upper zone reflects the number (w_R) and the fraction of responding cultures (F_+). The numerical values for PFC responses from individual wells are given on the x axis; the height of each 'step' on the y axis indicates the number of cultures with a given number of PFC. The central arrow refers to the median[**] value.

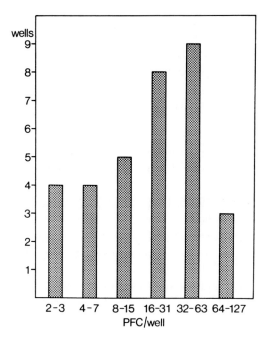

Figure 7.7. 'Grouped plot' presentation of the data used for clone size calculation

---

[**] Median is a value in an ordered set of values below and above which there is an equal number of values (*Webster's Ninth New Collegiate Dictionary*).

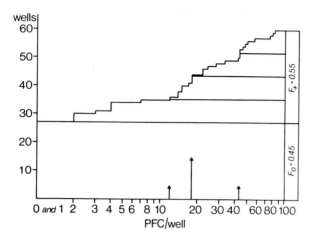

Figure 7.8. 'Cumulative plot' of the data obtained from a PFC assay of individual microcultures. Lower zone indicates the fraction of nonresponding cultures (F_0), upper zone the fraction of responding cultures (F_+). Ranked PFC values from individual microcultures are given on the x axis, the height of each 'step' on the y axis indicates the number of cultures with a given number of PFC. The central arrow refers to the median value. Interquartile range is delineated by smaller arrows

The interquartile ranges (enclosing the 50% most common values) are delineated by smaller arrows (the 25th and 75th percentile), and are an indication of the spread of responses observed.

Median is a good measure for a response when we intend to neglect the contribution of outlying values. The interquartile range is a good indication for homogeneity of the response.

The data given in the previous section (and already shown in the 'grouped plot' in Figure 7.7) are used for construction of the 'cumulative plot' (Figure 7.8). First we rank the values:

25x0, 1, 1, 2, 2, 2, 3, 4, 4, 4, 7, 12, 14, 14, 15, 15, 17, 18, 18, 18, 22, 22, 24, 28, 33, 42, 43, 43, 43, 46, 48, 50, 57, 76, 80, 83.

The 25 zeros and the two ones are considered as negatives. This forms the lower zone of the plot. The remaining 33 values are plotted step by step. The 17th value (from either side) is 18 PFC, and this is the *median*.

The 25th and 75th percentiles are the middle values between 0 – median and median – 100. The interquartile range is 12-43 PFC. The most common 50% of values is thus in the range of 12-43 PFC.

8 Lymphocyte functions resolved by LDA: a perspective

In this chapter we will provide the reader with data from a number of published experimental systems to indicate how the principles of LDA may be applied to the study of lymphocyte functions. Many of these examples represent a historical record, yet remain valuable today for experimental analyses as well as for understanding disease processes (see Chapter 9) and providing guides to therapy.

There are hundreds of publications on the use of LDA for studying lymphocyte function, and it is beyond the scope of this monograph to evaluate the published work exhaustively. The reader will find a more complete account of the relevant experiments on the website of this volume.

8.1 Measurement of B-cell frequencies

Limiting dilution analysis was first applied in immunology to provide frequency estimates of antigen-specific B cells. The strategy used was based on a rapid and sensitive detection system using haemolysis in agarose with antibody and complement. Any culture well containing a clone of cells producing antibody could be scored by yielding a haemolytic spot. Using this approach frequency estimates were obtained for B cells able to make antibody to sheep erythrocytes (SRBC) (Figure 8.1 and Appendix). In these studies B cells had to be activated either by using a polyclonal activator such as lipopolysaccharide (LPS), or by adding antigen (SRBC) together with some source of T-helper cells in excess. The frequency estimates ranged from 1×10^{-4} to 1×10^{-5}.

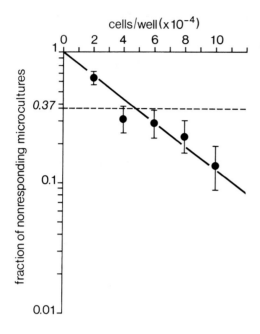

Figure 8.1. Demonstration of a single-hit curve. Titration of B cells. All microcultures contained a constant number of helper cells (2×10^4 per micro-culture). Spleen cells from nude mice were included as a source of B cells. Irradiated (fillers) and nonir-radiated (active) nude mouse spleen cells were mixed in different ratios to give 1.8×10^5 cells/well

8.2   Demonstration of multi-target events in the response to hapten–protein conjugates

Lymphocytes from mice primed to a hapten-carrier (TNP-KLH) are competent to make strong secondary immune responses *in vitro*. When lymphocytes from these animals were examined for the frequency of hapten-reactive cells then it emerged (Figure 8.2 and Appendix 1) that the titration curves that one obtained were more akin to multi-target curves than to single hit. This suggested that there were at least two populations of cells required for the responses, and that neither was in excess. In retrospect the result was not surprising as it emerged that the functional frequencies of T-helper cells and B cells were similar within the population.

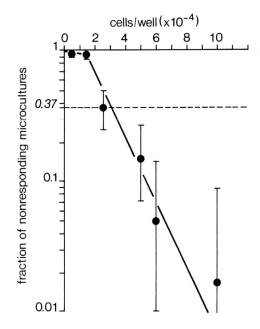

Figure 8.2. Demonstration of a multi-target curve. Titration of TNP-KLH-primed spleen cells for responses to TNP-KLH (1 µg/ml). All cell numbers were reconstituted to 1×10^5/well by addition of irradiated ATxBM spleen cells as fillers. 60 wells were sampled to provide data for each point

8.3 Estimating B-cell clone sizes

When B cells are triggered under limiting dilution conditions, some of the responding cultures will contain single clones, others will contain multiple clones. Clone size estimates of antibody-producing cells (PFC) were obtained by totalling the number of PFC (ΣPFC) from whole microculture trays (e.g. containing 60 culture wells), and dividing this by the number of precursors (n) calculated to be present in the whole plate – a value derived from the estimate of frequency. The mathematical background is given in sections 5.8 and 7.7.

A series of experiments of this kind suggested that clone sizes for thymus-independent (TI) antigens were generally less than those for T-dependent antigens (half to a third). In part this reflects the time required to reach the peak response for these different antigen categories, where the optimal T-dependent response often peaked 1-2 days after the TI response. For T-dependent antigens the larger clone sizes may have also reflected control by multiple cytokines with distinct growth and/or differentiation properties, whereas for TI antigens

control of clone size was more a feature of the initial B cell-activating properties of the antigen in question.

8.4 Clonal inactivation by high doses of thymus-independent (TI) antigens

The first demonstration that LDA could be used to monitor the loss of precursors in tolerance was that of Desaymard and Waldmann (1976). High doses of
TI antigens resulted in reduced antibody responses. LDA analysis showed that
this could be wholly accounted for by a reduced number of precursors engaged
in the response. Any precursor that produced a clone did so with clone sizes
comparable to those of non-tolerant cells. Comparison of precursor frequencies
to study the consequences of a tolerance-promoting encounter with antigen has
since been widely used as an experimental tool for both B- and T-lymphocyte
biology.

8.5 Evidence for existence of two types of T-helper cells

Once tissue culture methodology supportive of T–B cooperation had been
developed in the 1970s, the opportunity arose to analyse how T cells provide
help to B cells. The problem was not an easy one, as the frequencies of the
interacting cells were very low, and one needed experimental systems that
could accommodate this. Studies in large (bulk) cultures had shown that once
T cells had been primed *in vivo* with an antigen such as KLH, then two distinct
types of helper-memory response could be elicited. These were referred to by
various jargon terms, but two that caught on (at least in the USA!) were *cognate
and non-cognate recognition*. In the first case the molecular source of the epitope
that the T cell recognised needed to be the same as the one the B cell recognised
(reflecting the *in vivo* requirement for carrier and hapten to be linked). In the
second case the T-cell epitope could be expressed on a molecule distinct from
that to which the B cells were responding, giving rise to what was sometimes
referred to as *bystander* help. The question arose as to whether cognate and
non-cognate help were a function of similar or distinct T-cell subsets. Limiting
dilution and partition analysis helped to resolve this problem, suggesting the
latter as the answer.

8.5.1 Comparison of the frequencies of T cells providing cognate and non-cognate help

A way of obtaining T-cell populations primed to antigen was to 'educate' thymocytes by transferring them to irradiated recipients and then challenging
these animals with antigen (say SRBC or KLH). These T cells (T_{SRBC} or T_{KLH})
taken a week later as a highly enriched population, were referred to as 'educated' T cells. When T_{SRBC} were tested for their ability to help a constant

number of B cells (1×10^5/well) from adult-thymectomized, irradiated and bone marrow-reconstituted (ATxBM) mice, it was observed that the frequency of T-helper cells capable of helping SRBC responses was similar to that providing bystander help to the non-cross-reacting antigen DRBC (Figure 8.3). This suggested that educated T cells primed in this way were competent to offer non-cognate help. Actually this experiment was technically informative because the frequency of B cells responding to DRBC was less than that for SRBC, and resulted in 'levelling off in the readout'. The levelling off phenomenon required mathematical modifications to properly calculate frequency.

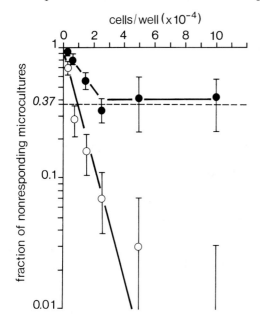

Figure 8.3. Frequencies of T cells providing cognate and non-cognate help. Titration of T_{SRBC} on the anti-SRBC and anti-DRBC responses to ATxBM spleen cells. The input of ATxBM cells was 1×10^5/well. All cultures contained 50 µl/ml of 1% SRBC and 50 µl/ml of 1% DRBC. Each point is based on spot test from 180 microcultures performed on day 5 of culture. (O) Spot test on SRBC. (●) Spot test on DRBC.(Taken from Waldmann *et al.*, 1975)

If T_{KLH} were taken from mice primed with soluble KLH alone, then one could compare the number of T cells helping cognate responses by using TNP-KLH (and TNP-primed B cells), and make a comparison with the number helping in a non-cognate way to the bystander antigen SRBC. We observed that T cells from animals primed without adjuvant had a high frequency of helpers of the non-cognate type, with absence of any helpers of the cognate type. When Freund's adjuvant was used in the priming protocol, then the frequency of non-cognate T-helper cells remained similar, but that of cognate T-helper cells was also high. This lack of correlation suggested the existence of two functionally distinct subsets of T cells.

This conclusion was further strengthened by the observation showing a lack of coincidence of responses to TNP (cognate) and SRBC (non-cognate) under limiting T-helper cell conditions. Using irradiated T-helper cells from mice primed with KLH in adjuvant, it was possible to show that the two readout responses (TNP and SRBC) segregated independently, suggesting that T-helper cells responsible for cognate and non-cognate help were themselves assorting independently (Table 8.1) (Waldmann and Pope, 1977; Marrack and Kappler, 1975).

Table 8.1. Rare coincidence between specific and nonspecific effects of T cells

		anti-SRBC [i]		
		+	−	
anti-TNP[ii]	+	34	39	73
	−	104	183	287
		138	222	360

[i] By spot test on duplicate SRBC plates

[ii] By plaque assay onto TNP-DRBC.

(Taken from Waldmann *et al.*, 1976a)

8.6 What is the effect of non-cognate help on B-cell function?

Work from bulk cultures had shown that T cells primed to KLH could release, into the medium, biologically active molecules capable of helping B-cell responses to the bystander antigen SRBC. It seemed important that the bystander antigen be particulate – probably a reflection of a signalling requirement for B cells (i.e. multivalent triggering) – so that they could benefit from the helper factors from T cells. A more suitable source of such T-helper cells and the factors they produce proved to be T cells stimulated by concanavalin A (Con A). Surprisingly the frequency of T-helper cells producing the panoply of factors required to promote a bystander response was around 1:19 000 of a naïve spleen population, suggesting that these cells are especially gifted or perhaps experienced to some unknown environmental antigen.

We questioned whether the, then unknown, factors could activate SRBC-specific B cells into proliferation or whether they were simply required for their differentiation into antibody secretion (as had been shown by Hünig *et al.*,

1974). LDA analyses of B cells exposed to T-helper supernatants for various lengths of time showed that help came from both events (enhanced proliferation and secretion). B cells exposed to SRBC and the 'factors' underwent rounds of division that were measurable as an increase in frequency of responsive B cells (Figure 8.4).

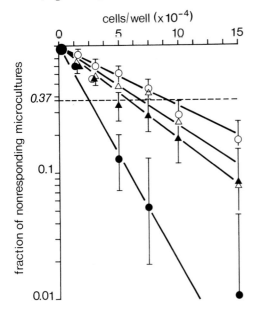

Figure 8.4. Increase in precursor frequency after exposure to antigen and helper factors. Titration of nude spleen cells for antibody responses after the following treatment. A 48 h exposure of nude spleen cells in preincubation with DRBC alone; (○) DRBC response, (▲) SRBC response. A 48 h exposure of nude spleen cells in preincubation with DRBC in the presence of Con A supernatant; (●) DRBC response, (△) SRBC response. Cells were redistributed and rechallenged with SRBC and DRBC in the presence of optimal help. Each point represents the result of 120 microcultures. (Taken from Waldmann *et al.*, 1976b)

In a series of replica plating studies (Figures. 8.5–8.7) it also emerged that there was much variability in the quality of biological activity arising from each individual non-cognate T-helper cell. Individual SRBC-specific B cells seemed differentially susceptible to the products of single T-helper cells, unlike their behaviour with the 'pooled' products from a bulk culture. We then predicted a heterogeneity of B cells, and a multiplicity of 'factors' influencing B-cell growth and differentiation.

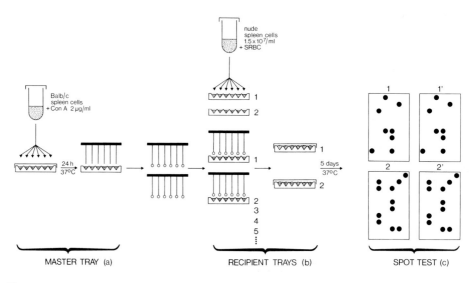

Figure 8.5. Flow diagram for the replica sampling experiment. (a) BALB/c spleen cells were mixed with Concanavalin A (final concentration 2 μg/ml) and dispensed in 15 μl volumes at 1 x 10⁴, 3 x 10⁴, 1 x 10⁵ cells/well in each of the three Terasaki trays and cultured for 24 h at 37°C. (b) Subsequently 1 μl samples from each well of the master trays were transferred into recipient trays containing 1.5 x 10⁵ nude spleen cells/well and antigen (SRBC). The manoeuvre was repeated eight times, such that eight parallel recipient trays were established from each master tray, and the recipient trays were cultured for five days at 37°C. (c) The haemolytic spot test was used to detect antibody to the antigen SRBC. (Taken from Lefkovits and Waldmann, 1977a, b)

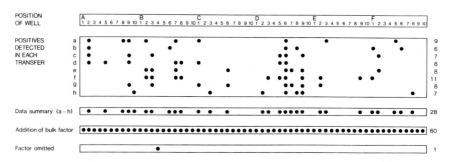

Figure 8.6. Results of the spot test of the eight recipient trays derived from a single master tray. The lines (a) – (h) refer to the recipient trays derived from the master tray containing 1 x 10⁴ BALB/c spleen cells/well. (The displays for the master trays of other cell concentrations are not presented.) The data summary incorporates all positive responses (●). Also shown are the results obtained from nude spleen cells cultured with helper factors from bulk cultures (positive control) or with normal medium (negative control). The position of a well in a master tray is defined by A-F, 1-10. (Taken from Lefkovits and Waldmann, 1977b)

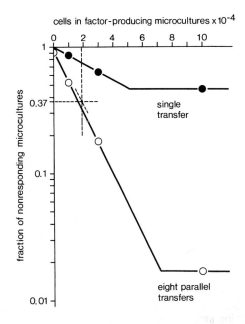

Figure 8.7. Titration of factor-producing cells in the master trays. (●) Titration curve based on a single transfer (the mean of scores from eight recipient wells); (○) titration curve based on the contribution of *all* eight parallel transfers. At F_0 = 0.37, the frequency of factor-producing cells (after correction for the background) was estimated as 1 in 19 000. (Taken from Lefkovits and Waldmann, 1977b)

Since that time there has, of course, been a resolution of those 'factors', now known as 'cytokines', produced by the T-helper cells, and of the heterogeneity that exists in B-cell subsets. We could now interpret our old data as saying that a positive B-cell response could only be elicited if a proper combination of cytokines complementary to the appropriate differentiation state of a given B cell were present in any particular responding well. The cytokines would include IL-2, IL-4 and IL-5, amongst others.

A significant lesson from this whole exercise is that the use of *replica plating of unknown biological activities from single T cells* can be a valuable procedure for assessing the complexity of interactions by products of single cells on target cells which are affected by them.

8.7   Cognate helper interactions

In this section we will describe the use of LDA to explore some of the properties of T-helper cells measurable in systems of linked recognition (i.e. situations where T cells recognise carrier epitopes and B cells recognise the hapten). At the time these studies began there was a significant literature accumulating (now disregarded but never retracted!) that cognate help operated through T-helper cells producing antigen-specific factors that provided all relevant biological activity necessary for B-cell growth and differentiation. This early literature distracted attention from other seemingly less exciting findings (e.g. helper cytokines and the growing evidence for genetic restriction of T–B cooperation). It seemed to us that LDA could help us to find out whether cooperation worked through widely diffusible antigen-specific T-cell factors or through direct T–B cell contact. The proposition could be tested by asking whether a single T-helper cell could cooperate with more than one B cell at any one time. By irradiating the T-helper cell we could retain helper function but avoid the generation of further progeny competent to cooperate. By presenting the single T cell with numerous antigen-specific B cells we could then test the question. We reasoned that if a T cell could cooperate by release of widely diffusible antigen-specific factors, as others had claimed, then the number should be greater than one. To our surprise, however, when we did the experiment, the answer was that cognate-type T-helper cells were monogamous.

The evidence was as follows.

(i)   The burst size of plaque-forming cells (PFC) supported by a single T cell was equivalent to that produced by a single B-cell clone. The experiment was performed such that we measured the total PFC (ΣPFC) for a whole culture tray (60 microcultures) at each input of T cells. From the fraction of negative wells for each tray, we derived the value for μ_{Th}. This value multiplied by 60 (the number of replicates per tray [i.e. per group]) gives an approximation of the number of functional T cells per culture tray of 60 wells. The ratio ΣPFC/total functional T cells gives the 'burst' size (Table 8.2). A range of experiments gave the burst size for a T-helper cell as 15-30 PFC, which was also the range for the B-cell clone size calculated in the same way (Waldmann *et al.*, 1976a).

Table 8.2. Burst size supported by a single Th cell

	T cells added	ΣPFC/60 wells	Estimates of μ	ΣPFC/total T$_{KLH}$
Exp. 1	1×10^5	5002	4.6	18.9
	5×10^4	2875	2.3	20.8
	2.5×10^4	1647	1.2	22.8
	1.25×10^4	416	0.4	17.3
	6.25×10^3	365	0.38	16.0
	none	21	–	–

Table 8.2 cont. Burst size supported by a single Th cell

	T cells added	ΣPFC/60 wells	Estimates of μ	ΣPFC/total T_{KLH}
Exp. 2	7.1×10^4	4097	4.2	17
	3.55×10^4	2530	2.12	19.9
	1.8×10^4	1415	1.04	22.6
	1.1×10^4	708	0.56	21.1
	7×10^3	589	0.47	21.9
	3.5×10^3	596	0.28	33.1
	none	0	–	–

(Waldmann, unpublished data)

(ii) Using plaque morphology, which could distinguish turbid from clear plaques, we observed that, where T-cell input was limiting, the number of positive wells showing a restricted morphological plaque type vs. heterogeneous (multiple) plaque types was high. In contrast, at saturating T-cell input the number of positive wells demonstrating 'multiples' was high. As the assay was designed on the basis that plaque morphology had a clonal basis, we were entitled to conclude that one T-helper cell probably cooperated with only a single B cell (Table 8.3).

Table 8.3. The relationship of T-cell input to the number of B-cell clones generated[i]

Input of T cells per microculture	Fraction of negative cultures[ii]	Number of wells containing single clones		Number of wells containing more than one clone[iii]	
		Observed	Expected	Observed	Expected
Nil	0.93	2	2.0	0	0
1.25×10^4	0.5	12	10.5	3	4.5
5×10^4	0.2	11	10.0	13	12.0
1×10^5	0.1	9	7.0	18	20.0

[i] 1.5×10^5 anti-Θ-treated TNP-FGG-primed spleen cells; 5 μg/ml TNP-KLH added to each well

[ii] Thirty microcultures sampled

[iii] Determined by plaque morphology

(Taken from Waldmann *et al.*, 1976a)

(iii) A more sophisticated procedure which clearly enumerated B-cell clones exploited isoelectric focusing of antibodies in the culture supernatants (Phillips and Waldmann, 1977). The basis of this was that a single B-cell clone would produce a single isoelectric spectrotype. In the absence of T cells we could see no antibody at all. In the presence of high numbers of T-helper cells we could see multiple spectrotype (i.e. clones) per well. In the presence of limiting T-helper cells most positive wells showed only a single spectrotype. We counted the total number of clonal products (spectrotypes) in this group and observed 66 spectrotype patterns from a total of 59 culture wells. We hypothesised that these B-cell products were the result of 1 T-cell : 1 B-cell interaction. In which case the B-cell clone numbers would be expected to segregate in the wells according to a Poisson distribution of T cells. Table 8.4 shows that the fit is very close ($\chi^2 = 1.76$). Thus from these data most of the T-helper cells must have been cooperating with only a single antigen-specific B cell. The number of wells containing multiple spectrotypes could be accounted for statistically by the chance distribution of multiple T cells into individual wells.

Table 8.4. Test of the hypothesis that a single T cell helps only one B cell

Number of clones	Number of wells which contain any given number of TNP-specific B cell-clones:	
	Observed	Expected
0	16	19.28
1	26	21.56
2	12	12.06
3	4	4.53
4	1	1.28
5	0	0.28

Analysis of the number of wells containing different numbers of B-cell clones from 59 samples. If we make the hypothesis that one T cell activates one B cell then the clones would be distributed according to the Poisson distribution of T cells getting into wells. A total number of 66 clones as observed would be expected to distribute as shown. (Taken from Phillips and Waldmann, 1977)

(iv) Finally, by using B cells where some were primed to the hapten NIP and others to TNP, we showed that a single T-helper cell (KLH-specific) could only give help to either a NIP-specific or a TNP-specific B cell even though it was confronted with many (Figure 8.8 and Table 8.5).

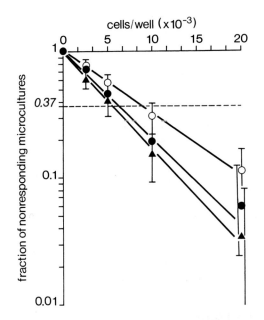

cells/well ($\times 10^{-3}$)

Figure 8.8. Titration of KLH-primed T cells on the response of TNP- and NIP-OVA-primed B spleen cells to NIP-KLH and TNP-KLH (1 μg/ml). A series of plots have been constructed assuming that the highest 0, 1.7%, 5% and 10% values of wells in the background (B cells alone) group were positive. Each point is based on the analysis of 60 to 120 samples. (Taken from Waldmann *et al.*, 1978)

The analysis is correct only if there is no ambiguity in scoring responding cells. Since there is always a certain background, limiting dilution data were plotted assuming that background responses might influence the readout. Figure 8.8 shows that whether or not noise is excluded made little difference to the single-hit nature of the curve or to the frequency estimates of KHL-specific T-helper cells.

Table 8.5. Observed and expected frequencies

		Observed			Expected (1T : 1B)				Expected (1T : 2B)		
		TNP				TNP				TNP	
		+	−			+	−			+	−
NIP	+	43	38	81	+	40.5	40.5	81	+	57.8	24.2	82
	−	17	22	39	−	19.5	19.5	39	−	5.6	32.5	38.1
		60	60	120		60	60	120		63.4	56.7	120.1
						$\chi^2 = 0.95$	df = I			$\chi^2 = 29.8$	df = I	

Not only did these experiments rule out the concept of widely diffusible factors, they suggested that T-helper cells formed monogamous relationships with B cells that persisted through the culture period. As we knew that the influence of T-helper cells is required for at least 4 days of the culture period, we surmised that there is a mechanism for retaining the influence of the Th cell in the vicinity of the growing clone. A possible mechanism for this is that there is some chemotactic factor (or chemokine) made by one or other of the T cell and B cell that ensures that each cell and its progeny remains confined to the very local microenvironment. Perhaps in that way the T cell is monogamous to the clone, but promiscuous with its members.

The current dogma on T–B cooperation accepts that contact must occur, and involves interaction of TCR with MHC class II-bound peptide, CD4 with MHC class II, CD28 with B7, CD40 ligand with CD40 and many others. The conclusion of cell contact in T–B cooperation was counter to dogma, and emerged during a dark and disreputable period of cellular immunology. It is indeed pleasing that the LDA data have held out so clearly in opposition to the fashion of that time.

8.8   Application of LDA to other T-cell functions

LDA has now been applied to the measurement of frequencies of many functions ascribed to T cells where those functions have had some clear-cut *in vitro* correlate. These include estimation of frequencies of T cells reacting to antigen by proliferation, release of cytokines, generation of cytotoxic T cells (pCTL) and very recently by even suppression of responses. Some of these assay systems have actually been applied clinically. The measurement of so-called precursors of CTL (or pCTL) has now been widely exploited as an indicator of histocompatibility over MHC class I differences, and consequently the risk of GVHD in marrow transplantation. Similarly, estimates of incompatibility of T cells across class II MHC has come from the calculation of T cells that can be activated to release cytokines such as IL-2 which promote CTL activity in a two-stage assay.

8.8.1   CTL assays

These were pioneered by three groups in the mid-1970s. Skinner and Marbook (1976) utilised polyacrylamide rafts with dimpled surfaces to segregate clones. Lindahl and Wilson (1977) and Teh *et al.*, (1977) adapted microtitre trays. Since that time measurements of pCTL have probably provided the major rationale for application of LDA in studies of transplantation compatibility, viral immunity and basic studies on immunological tolerance. The power of these systems was highlighted by studies of Teh *et al.* (1997) when they demonstrated that virtually all wells that exhibited primary killer activity could be re-stimulated to secondary CTL function, estimating the final clone sizes to be somewhere in the order of 1000 cells.

pCTL measurements in human are equally robust and since the first edition of this book these have become commonplace in the literature. They have gained a particular place in the assessment of potential donor–recipient combinations for unrelated allogeneic marrow transplantation where there would seem to be some useful correlation between the frequency of alloreactive cells and the risk of GVHD. Equally, in the assessment of the way the recipient of a transplant has adapted immunologically to the graft, there is some indication that lack of pCTL may be a partial indicator of immunological tolerance. Such information could help the transplant physician decide which patients might benefit from reduced immunosuppression (see Chapter 9).

8.8.2   LDA of T cells reactive to antigens and mitogens

The feasibility of using LDA to measure the frequencies of human peripheral blood T cells proliferating in response to antigens such as PPD and tetanus toxoid has been well demonstrated in the past (Van Oers *et al.*, 1978, 1979).

There have not, however, been many publications using LDA and proliferation assays, and it isn't entirely clear why this is. A thorough analysis of how to apply LDA to the proliferation capacity of murine cells emerges from publications of Chen and coworkers (1982) and Dozmorov and coworkers (1995a). The latter authors observed that CD4 T cells from old (but not young) mice showed non-linear dose–response curves when stimulated with the mitogen Con A. Not only were these responses nonlinear, but they were also graphically 'zig-zag'. The authors postulated and indeed obtained experimental evidence for the hypothesis that there was an abundant cell type with high proliferative potential (LPC1) and a less abundant inhibitory population with low proliferative potential (LPC2). At high T-cell input the proliferation of the abundant population was inhibited by the population with poor proliferative potential.

The mechanism by which the 'regulatory' population inhibits the LPC1 is unknown but could perhaps involve competition for growth factors or release of inhibitory cytokines such as IL-10. Why inhibitory cells should accumulate with age is unclear, but perhaps these represent the accumulation of cells tolerant to a wide range of self and nonself antigens. In terms of proliferation, these cells seem to behave as if anergic. In functional terms they would seem to interfere with growth of otherwise competent cells giving the appearance of being regulatory.

It may be that this is the first reliable measure of cells with regulatory potential *in vivo*, and perhaps sets the scene for how we might come to analyse T cells with suppressive function.

8.8.3   Suppressor T cells

There can be little doubt about the existence of T cells that regulate or suppress immune responses *in vivo*. Despite the abundance of *in vivo* data to support the existence of such cells, there is yet very little *in vitro* data, let alone LDA material to study their life-styles. There has been a tacit assumption with all T-cell functions that the relevant T cell should be grown as a line and then cloned.

This has never been demonstrated for T cells with consistently suppressive properties, other than in the context of Th1/Th2 immune deviation, although recently a new cell type called TR1 (T-regulatory cell 1) has been exposed as a potential candidate for the label of a T-suppressor cell.

The lack of *in vitro* data for Ts cells could be explained by any of the following possibilities:

(i)   that suppression/regulation is an *in vivo* phenomenon requiring specialised microenvironments that have not been established *in vitro*

(ii) that suppression is a feature of cells with low proliferative potential, and not amenable to this sort of analysis

(iii) that suppression is a multicellular population problem which cannot at present be reduced to single cell analysis.

8.9   Overview

LDA has and will continue to provide its own distinct form of information on T-cell behaviour. In modern-day immunology it is assumed that TCR transgenic mice now provide enriched populations of T cells with appropriate antigen specificity. It remains to be seen just how many of these T cells have the desired functions that can be measured by LDA. If there is functional heterogeneity, how will the sub-populations interact? Will suppression be visible or possible in a population with just a single T-cell receptor? We are sure that useful new information on these issues will emerge as LDA is coupled with the new technological approaches to cell function.

9 The clinical potential of LDA

9.1 Why have a clinical chapter?

The applications of immunology to clinical medicine have surprisingly not kept pace with rapid advances in the basic science. However, things are beginning to change, and the use of LDA and partition analysis may provide the clinician with new insights into disease processes, enable decisions to be taken on adjustments or withdrawal of therapy and may even provide quality control for new therapeutic approaches in areas such as transplantation, vaccination to microbial and tumour antigens and vaccine strategies aimed at inducing tolerance or 'reprogramming' the immune system in autoimmune disease.

In transplantation and in autoimmune diseases, our goals for the future are to provide short-term immunosuppressive therapy to achieve long-term therapeutic benefit. Current therapies penalise the whole of the immune system for the misdemeanours of very few of its lymphocytes, so risking infection and a range of other unwanted side-effects. Our goal should be to find therapeutic approaches that leave intact immunity to microbial pathogens, while ensuring tolerance to the target tissue.

LDA and partition analysis serve a purpose in providing information on the existence, frequency and functional phenotype of cells capable of responding to those target antigens, so permitting the clinician to select and manipulate the lymphocyte content of donor and recipient cells in transplantation, and to monitor the fate of host antigen reactive cells in autoimmunity. Accumulating databases which catalogue and correlate the influence of antigen-specific lymphocyte frequency with disease progression will eventually lead to routine use of LDA-based measures as diagnostics to tailor therapy both *in vivo* and *in vitro*.

Below we provide the reader with examples from the literature to show the progress that is being made.

9.2   Bone marrow transplantation

Bone marrow transplants (BMT) are performed to rescue a defective haemopoietic system. In most instances this arises in the treatment of leukaemia where supralethal chemo/radiotherapy is given to eradicate as much of the leukaemic mass as possible, with unavoidable damage to host stem cells. If the marrow transplant comes from a non-identical donor then there can be problems with contaminating donor T cells reacting against the host producing graft-versus-host disease (GVHD). This can be managed to some extent by providing strong immunosuppression with drugs. However, it seems more desirable to remove donor T cells from the graft as this is so easy to do.

In practice this does indeed reduce the incidence of GVHD, but leaves the patient deprived of T cells which will protect against infection. It also removes the extra benefit of the so-called graft-versus-leukaemia (GVL) effect, where alloreactive donor cells kill the residual leukaemic cells to enable a greater number of 'cures'.

Of the many strategies aimed at avoiding some of these complications, so as to enable BMT to be extended outside the family in so-called 'unrelated transplants', the simplest has been that of pre-selecting donors based on some clear measure of their potential for alloreactivity to recipient cells. A number of centres have attempted to correlate risk of GVHD with precursor frequency of CTL precursors (pCTL) or of T-helper cells (cells releasing IL-2 on stimulation by recipient cells). Although information is still accumulating, there is evidence that Th frequencies might be predictive of good matches. The predictive value of pCTL measures are less clear-cut, with some publications claiming utility and others not (Schwarer *et al.*, 1993, 1994; Bunjes *et al.*, 1995b; Montagna *et al.*, 1996; Hornick *et al.*, 1997).

The enthusiasm for T-cell depletion of bone marrow came with expectation that new T cells would develop in the recipient thymus. This expectation is met in children, but not in adults, where the thymus appears to lose its capacity to act as a high output primary lymphoid organ. The result is that T-cell reconstitution in the transplanted patient is very slow, and initially dependent on the few post-thymic T cells that were left. The challenge now is to find ways to speed up functional T-cell reconstitution so that the patient achieves normal immunity as soon as possible.

One approach is to seek a source of T cells which naturally lack the capacity to mediate GVHD. It has been suggested that blood from the umbilical cord of pooled random 'donors' may serve this purpose as *in vitro* responses in bulk cultures suggest diminished MLR and CTL potential. However, the results of LDA shows that high frequencies of pCTL and Th are present, which suggests that cord-blood may not provide the desired solution (Keever *et al.*, 1995).

Another, and more promising direction is to try and reconstitute the patient with T cells from the donor where all alloreactive (anti-recipient) T cells have been removed in an *in vitro* pre-incubation step. Donor cells incubated with recipient stimulators can be exposed to a variety of agents that either kill or tolerise the responding cells, leaving other T cells intact. In order to monitor the efficacy of the procedure, LDA of the starting and final preparations are required. Although these procedures have been tried and tested in animal models, they have yet to be applied in clinical practice. Almost certainly LDA will be required to validate the protocols, and to monitor the degree of depletion once these become routine.

The hope is that sufficient of these negatively selected T-cell populations will be transplanted to provide adequate anti-microbial immunity and some GVL potential (Bunjes *et al.*, 1995a).

LDA and partition analysis may also enable the clinician to investigate mechanisms of tolerance in the transplanted patients. Previous studies with haploidentical transplants have provided evidence that regulatory mechanisms may operate to limit alloreactivity in some cases (Rosenkrantz *et al.*, 1990).

9.3 Organ transplantation

Current practice in immunosuppression of patients receiving organ transplants is to maintain such patients on life-long immunosuppression. In some cases this may not be necessary as there are examples of patients that have discontinued immunosuppression, and yet do not reject their graft. It would therefore be desirable to have a means to select patients for whom gradual drug dose reduction and ultimately discontinuation could be achieved. Recent work of Batten *et al.* (1995) has compared by LDA the frequency of alloreactive cells (Th) in patients whose grafts had failed from acute rejection with those whose grafts failed for other reasons. They noticed low-to-absent donor-specific Th in 50% of the latter group, with normal reactivity to third party. No such difference was found in the patients who had rejected their kidney (Mason *et al.*, 1996). This finding may provide some basis for selecting patients for drug withdrawal.

Looking to the future we can expect immunosuppression to change towards using drugs or newer biological agents to promote allograft tolerance. Where tolerance is expected to operate by deletional mechanisms, then LDA will be necessary to monitor efficacy, before consideration of drug withdrawal. Where tolerance is expected to operate through regulatory mechanisms, then LDA and partition analysis may enable one to monitor the emergence of the desired regulatory cells on the basis of their capacity to inhibit the responses at high cell input, and on the basis of the cytokines or other cell-type-specific products that they make.

Due to the lack of donor organs it is predicted that the need for organs can only be met through xenotransplantation of pig organs to human. If the problem of hyperacute rejection through antibody can be solved, then the question arises as to what the strength of the cellular xenoreactive response will be. Dorling *et al.*, (1996) have used LDA to show that the total anti-pig response could even be stronger than the alloreactive (human vs. human) response, in particular that mediated through indirect processing of pig antigens. We can predict that if transplantation of pig organs does become the norm in organ grafting, then use of LDA will also be a critical part of the monitoring process in designing the best immunosuppressive strategies.

9.4   Monitoring the efficacy of vaccination and cellular immuno-therapy directed to viruses and cancer cells

9.4.1   The immunosuppressed host

There are many circumstances where one would like to be able to monitor the capacity of host T cells to react to defined viral and tumour antigens in assessing how best to enhance or maintain the targeted immune function.

In marrow transplantation there is a risk of Epstein–Barr virus-induced lymphoproliferative disease (EBV-LPD) during the first 6 months. This is correlated with a substantial deficiency of anti-EBV pCTL. Donor peripheral blood cell infusions can cause tumour regression by restoring high levels of pCTL to the host (Lucas *et al.*, 1996).

In the coming era, where more transplants will be performed in unrelated and MHC mismatched combinations, and where T-cell depletion of the donor marrow will be needed, it will be essential to ensure adequate anti-viral immunity through vaccination or donor cell infusions. LDA will be needed to establish the extent and duration of these immunologically based anti-viral strategies.

9.4.2   The longitudinal monitoring of anti-viral immunity

The long-term reproducibility of LDA performed on human peripheral blood cells in monitoring anti-viral immunity has been well demonstrated for varicella zoster by Hayward and colleagues (1994). By measuring frequencies of T cells producing Th1 and Th2-type cytokines it would seem that the capacity to produce γ-IFN wanes with age (Zhang *et al.*, 1994). This somewhat sophisticated use of LDA may have broader application for evaluating the efficacy of therapies designed to deviate the human immune response toward a more efficient protective immunity.

9.4.3   Uncovering immune potential where none was expected

Children born with vertically transmitted HIV seem to have far less CTL activity in their blood than adults. LDA suggests that the pCTL to various viral antigens are there, but that these cells have not received adequate stimulation to drive them to clonal proliferation and differentiation (McFarland *et al.*, 1994). Knowledge of their presence encourages attempts to improve HIV vaccination in this group of patients.

9.4.4 Testing new vaccine strategies

The advances in knowledge about how T cells become activated by antigen will increasingly lead to new vaccine strategies, which will require good quantitative measures of potency. For example, the introduction of the gene for human B7.1 to a vector carrying the surface antigen gene of hepatitis B resulted in a greater number of pCTL being generated than the viral antigen alone (He *et al*, 1996). Application of such 'smart' vaccines to humans will require similar quantitation by LDA to show their worth.

Use of comparable tumour vaccine strategies will equally require LDA to monitor the degree and duration of the host response (Arienti *et al.*, 1994).

9.5 Autoimmune disease

There are very few autoimmune diseases where all target antigens are known. However, for many diseases we do know at least some of the antigens. It is, however, surprising that only in multiple sclerosis have serious attempts been made to monitor the frequencies of autoreactive T cells (Brod *et al.*, 1991; Chou *et al.*, 1992; Satyanarayana *et al.*, 1993; Stinissen *et al.*, 1995; Bieganowska *et al.*, 1997). Partitioning of such cells in LDA-based culture systems may free them from inhibitory regulatory processes (e.g. activation-induced death through Fas/Fas-ligand interactions) and so permit them to be enumerated (Bieganowska *et al.*, 1997). The data suggest that a significant number of multiple sclerosis patients do have high frequencies of myelin basic protein-reactive T cells and that these could be monitored in evaluating new therapeutic strategies. LDA assays designed to follow the emergence and disappearance of T cells with particular functional phenotypes, may prove valuable in correlating remissions with T-cell behaviour.

This broad principle could be applied to any autoimmune disease with known autoreactivity to a defined antigen.

9.6 Applications to allergy

There are numerous examples of allergic diseases where the antigens are known, and desensitisation would be desirable. If it were possible to measure the frequencies of T cells of different functional phenotypes, and to correlate these with disease, then therapies could adjusted to deviate the response (Li *et al.*, 1994, 1996). This is exemplified in a study of allergic rhinitis to grass pollen (Li *et al.*, 1996). Patients who were highly atopic and those who had no allergic symptoms were compared for frequencies of CD4 T cells producing cytokines on stimulation with antigen. Surprisingly, the frequencies of such cells were equivalent between the two groups. However, the ratio of T cells producing γ-IFN and those making IL-4 were distinctly different between the groups (117:1 and 4:1), respectively.

This sort of non-invasive approach to monitoring allergic disease and its treatment could have broad application to asthma, rhinitis and insect- and drug-induced allergies.

9.7 Overview

Both short- and long-term assessments of the frequencies of antigen-reactive cells with different functional phenotypes will become an important diagnostic tool for monitoring disease progression and its therapeutic control. The vigilant observer may be able to examine the behaviour of cell populations subject to partition analysis and be able to focus on cells that inhibit or interfere with the response. This may provide a handle to measure regulatory cells which could be beneficial in many cases, or harmful in others. Once such cells become well defined, the measurement of their products may become possible, allowing calculation of the precursor frequencies of Ts (regulators) in their own right, and consequently correlation of their presence with disease processes.

At present the special value of LDA is to provide a longitudinal measure of events within the individual patient. Eventually, as techniques become more refined and standard protocols adopted by different clinical centres, we can expect a definition of 'normals' and 'abnormals' in particular disease settings. At that point LDA will have a clear place in decisions for patient care made by the physician.

10 LDA program

Two diskettes are included in the pocket at the back of this monograph. The installation procedure for the software package is given on the page facing the diskette pocket.

In this chapter the use of the LDA program is described, while in chapter 11 a description of the LDA simulation program is given. The two software components are linked, so that data from the simulation experiments can be treated in the LDA program as if they had been obtained by bench work.

This software package provides all the necessary calculation procedures and plotting tools for performing evaluations of limiting dilution analyses:

(i)   it provides a customised spreadsheet into which the results of limiting dilution experiments are entered

(ii)   it draws a semi-log plot

(iii) it draws a linear regression line

(iv) it calculates the frequency of the precursor cells

(v)   it calculates the chi-square values and estimates the p values

(vi) it calculates and draws 95% confidence limits

(vii) it prepares printouts of a quality suitable for publication

Theoretical aspects are dealt with in relevant chapters.

10.1   Dilutions and treatments

The program can be opened by clicking either on the LDA icon or on any previously saved file of an actual experiment (see also section 10.9).

Upon opening the program a dialog box appears:

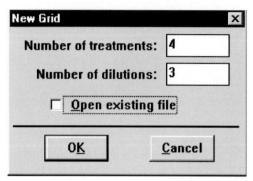

and the user is asked to enter the number of treatments and the number of dilutions he intends to perform.

If he uses a single type of suspension and induces the response at three different concentrations of antigen, and in one control without added antigen, he chooses 4 *treatments*.

If he wants to perform the experiment at three different cell inputs (5000, 20 000, 50 000 cells/well) he will choose 3 *dilutions*.

Upon confirming OK, the window **Noname 1** appears (see next page). As will become clear later, each new experiment receives a consecutive number (**Noname 2, Noname 3**...). The experiment can later be saved under this name or any name the user chooses (see section 10.9).

10.2   Layout of the LDA window

The window is divided into three areas:

(i)   data area (spreadsheet for data entry; the size of the table depends on the number of treatments and number of dilutions)

(ii)   plot, called by default **Noname 1, Noname 2, Noname 3**, etc. (and sequentially numbered until the experiment is saved or discarded)

(iii) calculation area on which all the computer calculations (frequencies, 95% confidence limits, chi-square) are shown

The size of any of the areas can be altered by dragging the area separator. (The consequence of changing portions of the window is illustrated in section 10.6).

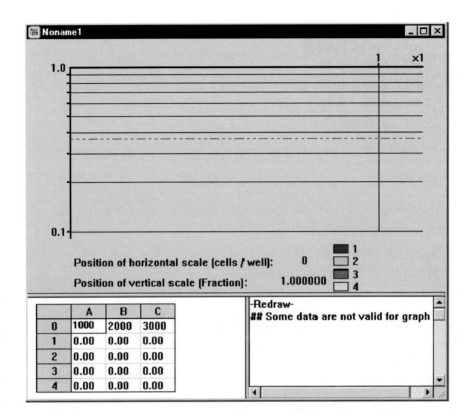

10.3 Spreadsheet for data entry

The spreadsheet for 3 dilutions and 4 treatments has the following format:

	A	B	C
0	1000	2000	3000
1	0.00	0.00	0.00
2	0.00	0.00	0.00
3	0.00	0.00	0.00
4	0.00	0.00	0.00

The first line of the spread sheet (labelled '0') is reserved for cell input per well. In the first step of entering data, the user must replace the default values 1000, 2000 and 3000 with the chosen input.

Let the user choose 5000, 20 000 and 50 000 cells per well.

	A	B	C
0	5000	20000	50000
1	0.00	0.00	0.00
2	0.00	0.00	0.00
3	0.00	0.00	0.00
4	0.00	0.00	0.00

10.4   Responding or nonresponding cultures

The experimenter now has to decide whether he wishes to enter the data as

- the number of nonresponding cultures
- the fraction of nonresponding cultures
- the number of responding cultures
- the fraction of responding cultures

This is done by choosing **Settings** in the sub-menu **Graph.**

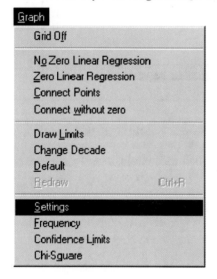

The box **Settings** appears on which the experimenter is expected to choose whether he will record the data in the form of responding or nonresponding cultures.

The usual choice (in the frame **Select fraction**) is:

◉ *Nonresponding*

Obviously another option is:

◉ *Responding.*

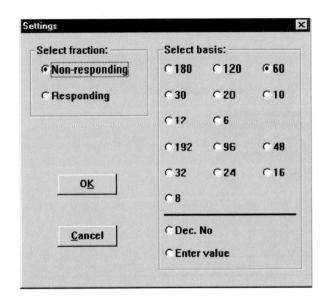

Whatever the choice, the program needs to know the number of micro-cultures used for each experimental point, so the user activates the appropriate number in the frame **Select basis**. It should be noted that the first three lines (8 choices) refer to Terasaki trays (their multiples/fractions), while the bottom three lines (7 choices) refer to microtitre plates (their multiples/fractions). If values other than those indicated are expected to be used, the value of the number of wells can be entered by selecting

◉ *Enter value*

Note that whatever the choice, the program calculates the fraction of *non-responding* cultures.

The above procedure is valid for most experimental conditions. It fails when not all experimental points are based on the same number of wells (for example when 60 cultures were used, but there was a contamination in one tray, and say six cultures had to be discounted [leaving 54 experimental cultures]). In a case such as this, one should enable

◉ *Dec. No.*

Instead of 22 nonresponding cultures one enters the value 0.407 (22 non-responding cultures out of 54).

Using this option, the calculation of 95% confidence limits might yield false results. It is recommended to stick to one option throughout the experiment. Fortunately, inapplicable entries are immediately detected by 'out-of-scale' graphs. In such instances the 'settings' have to be altered accordingly, and clicking on **Redraw** will provide correct plots.

For the example given here, the user will now choose:

◉ *Nonresponding*

and

Select basis: ◉ 60 wells

Note that if one enters the fraction of cultures rather than the actual number, the user will be asked to indicate how many cultures were tested (this dialog box will appear when the confidence limit calculation is requested).

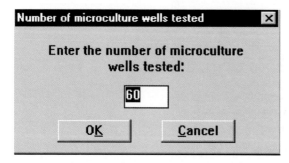

10.5   Linear regression

Let us assume that for the four titrations the experimenter obtained these results:

	A	B	C
0	5000	20000	50000
1	55	30	10
2	55	22	0
3	57	57	58
4	60	10	1

We should remember that each entry on the spreadsheet (rows 1-4) represents the number of *non-responding* cultures. The program calculates the F_0 values (55/60, 30/60, 10/60, etc.) which then appear on the plot.

In the sub-menu **Graph** he clicks on **Redraw,** upon which four titration curves appear.

The straight lines represent linear regression by 'least square method'. The calculation is performed in such a way that only the experimental points are considered in the calculation, and the *origin* (the zero point of the cell input) is neglected.

Note that the four lines are colour-coded (line 1 is dark blue, line 2 green, line 3 red and line 4 is light blue). The colour coding will be dealt with in section 10.9.

Linear regression through the experimental points:

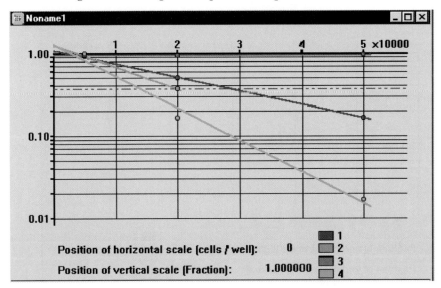

If it is assumed (and in many instances it is) that the curve has to pass through the origin, then this option can be activated in the submenu **Graph**. The justification of one or another option is given in the relevant chapters of the LDA monograph.

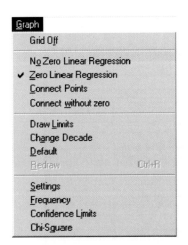

Note that line 2 (green) connects only to cell input 20 000, since the next entry, for 50 000 cells, is disregarded from the plot (see p. 153 of this section) Line 3 (red) coalesces with the x axis. Typically, this type of titration curve is obtained for negative control (e.g. antigen omitted).

Linear regression through the origin:

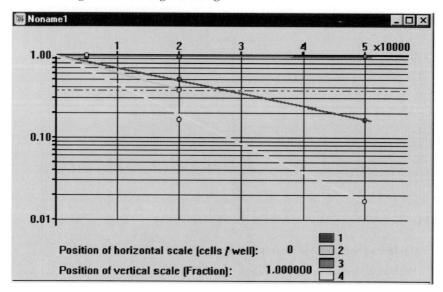

There are two other options for the graphical display, both allowing points to be connected. In some instances one wishes to connect only the experimental points, in other ones all points including the *origin*. Again these options are selectable in the sub-menu **Graph**.

Plot connecting the experimental points:

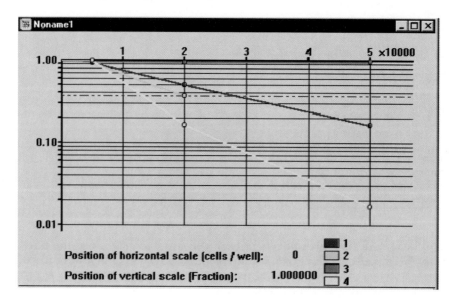

The user should be aware of the fact that if the titration contains the result 'zero' (in this experiment treatment 2, dilution C), this point is disregarded in the graphical representation, since zero cannot be plotted on the log scale. The user has the option to 'Consider 0 as 1 nonresponding culture'.

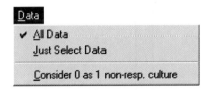

This option is used in instances when omitting an entire data set (60 responding cultures) would distort the results to a larger extent than when one assumes that 59 instead of 60 cultures responded. Activating the above option does not alter the tabulated values (*does not replace* 0 with 1), but *considers* the zeros as 1 for the plot.

10.6   Frequency calculations

For the linear regression lines (through origin or not) the frequency calculations are performed by choosing **Frequency** in the sub-menu **Graph**.

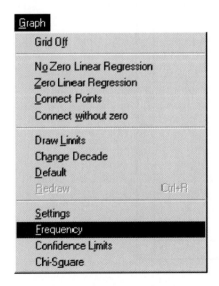

The results of the estimates are presented in the calculation area.

For display purposes the calculation area was increased by dragging the area separator. As an alternative the data area is kept small and the data are inspected by scrolling. All data can be exported and kept as protocols.

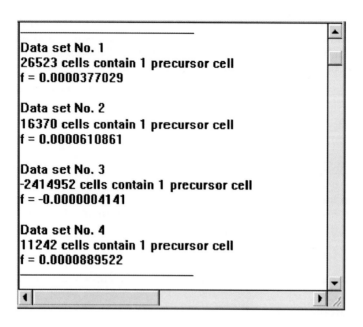

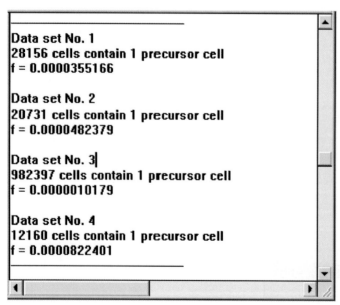

Note that for the two options (through origin or not) separate frequency calculations are performed. In the above example there are eight values, the first set referring to the linear regression disregarding the origin, the second set linear regression through the origin.

10.7   Confidence limits

In the next step, confidence limits are calculated and displayed.

In sub-menu **Graph** in two consecutive steps one chooses **Confidence Limits** and **Draw Limits**. The calculation area now displays the numerical values, and the graph incorporates the 95% bars (if they do not show, the user should click in the sub-menu **Graph** on **Redraw**).

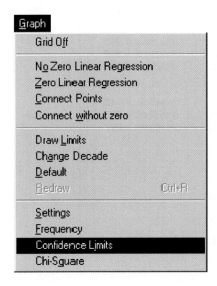

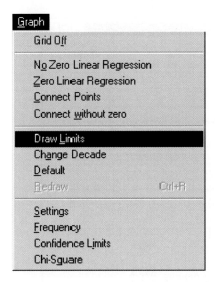

The calculation area shows the computed values:

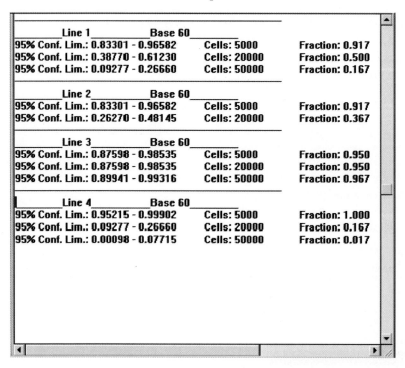

```
          Line 1              Base 60
95% Conf. Lim.: 0.83301 - 0.96582      Cells: 5000       Fraction: 0.917
95% Conf. Lim.: 0.38770 - 0.61230      Cells: 20000      Fraction: 0.500
95% Conf. Lim.: 0.09277 - 0.26660      Cells: 50000      Fraction: 0.167

          Line 2              Base 60
95% Conf. Lim.: 0.83301 - 0.96582      Cells: 5000       Fraction: 0.917
95% Conf. Lim.: 0.26270 - 0.48145      Cells: 20000      Fraction: 0.367

          Line 3              Base 60
95% Conf. Lim.: 0.87598 - 0.98535      Cells: 5000       Fraction: 0.950
95% Conf. Lim.: 0.87598 - 0.98535      Cells: 20000      Fraction: 0.950
95% Conf. Lim.: 0.89941 - 0.99316      Cells: 50000      Fraction: 0.967

          Line 4              Base 60
95% Conf. Lim.: 0.95215 - 0.99902      Cells: 5000       Fraction: 1.000
95% Conf. Lim.: 0.09277 - 0.26660      Cells: 20000      Fraction: 0.167
95% Conf. Lim.: 0.00098 - 0.07715      Cells: 50000      Fraction: 0.017
```

while the plot contains the relevant graphical representation of the confidence limits.

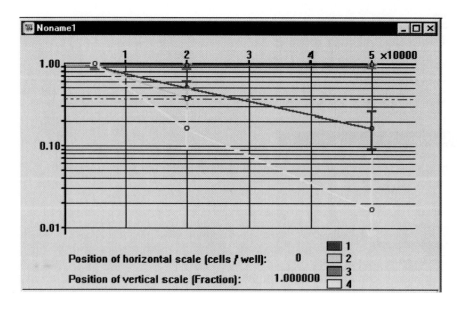

The user should note that the 95% confidence limit values are correct for any choice of up to 171 cultures. Because of the 'overflow' of the factorials above 171!, the confidence limits for higher numbers of cultures are erroneous.

10.8 Chi-square

Linear regression yields a straight line regardless of the quality of the data. A type of quality control exists which enables the user to check if the fit of the data to a straight line is acceptable or not. The test is named 'chi-squared test for goodness of fit' and involves the calculation of chi-square values and a judgement on whether or not the experimental data fit the regression line. This is done by calculating the chi-square values. Again in the sub-menu **Graph** one has to click on **Chi-Square** and in the calculation area the chi-square value appears.

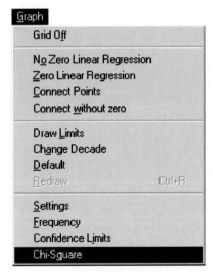

In principle, low chi-square indicates good fit, high chi-square bad fit. p values below 0.05 suggest that the hypothesis that the computed regression line is a good model for the data should be rejected. The actual chi-square and p values are displayed in the calculation area.

The reader is urged to consult sections 4.3, 4.4 and Appendix/5 in order to ensure that he interprets the results correctly and that he chooses the proper conditions under which the 'null hypothesis' is accepted or rejected.

```
┌──────────────────────────────────┬──┐
│ ─────────────────────            │▲ │
│ Data set No. 1                   │  │
│ Chi-Square 0.185   p = 1.00000   │  │
│                                  │  │
│ Data set No. 2                   │  │
│ Chi-Square 0.000   p = 1.00000   │  │
│                                  │  │
│ Data set No. 3                   │  │
│ Chi-Square 0.026   p = 1.00000   │  │
│                                  │  │
│ Data set No. 4                   │  │
│ Chi-Square 13.028  p = 0.00150   │  │
│                                  │  │
│ ─────────────────────            │  │
│ Data set No. 1                   │  │
│ Chi-Square 2.795   p = 0.39163   │  │
│                                  │  │
│ Data set No. 2                   │  │
│ Chi-Square 6.165   p = 0.04979   │▓ │
│                                  │  │
│ Data set No. 3                   │  │
│ Chi-Square 27.018  p = 5.887e-006│  │
│                                  │  │
│ Data set No. 4                   │  │
│ Chi-Square 30.786  p = 8.500e-007│▼ │
├──────────────────────────────────┼──┤
│ ◄ │                       │ ►   │  │
└──────────────────────────────────┴──┘
```

It is not within the scope of this chapter to provide data interpretations for the displayed examples. Nevertheless it should be noted that the data set No. 2 is based on 2 experimental points, the linear regression line coinciding with those points, and therefore the chi-square equals zero.

A chi-square versus p value chart is given in section 2 of the Appendix.

10.9   Log grid, colours of the line and saving the data

The user has an option to switch the logarithmic grid on or off. This is done in sub-menu **Graph** by clicking on **Grid On** or **Grid Off**.

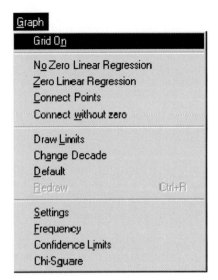

The graph can be displayed at one or more decades (logarithmic ranges). The choice of the decades is of importance if one wishes to keep one format for several experiments (if data are displayed which are all within one decade, the plot will also be of one decade); the user might want to use two decades, and he can do so by clicking in the sub-menu **Graph** on **Change Decade**.

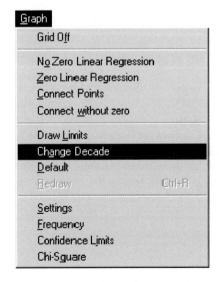

The colour of the line can be chosen or altered by double clicking on the small square next to the numbers 1, 2, ... on the semi-log plot. Upon this action the colour palette appears.

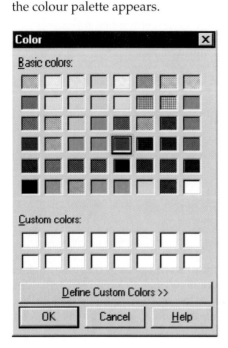

Any colour can be chosen. Since the choice will also dictate the outcome of the quality print (see below), we recommend choosing black if a 'black and white' print is intended (this is of course the case in most instances), or a bright colour for a slide or colour print.

The experiment can be saved (**File** menu) by giving the experiment a name followed by extension **.lda**; e.g. KLHstim1.lda. When starting the program next time, one opens the file for any chosen experiment.

Note that on the x and y axes horizontal and vertical bars are superimposed. These can be dragged to any position of the graph. This provides the reader with the opportunity to explore the plots, e.g. to indicate the slopes. When the bars are dragged, the numbers 0 and 1.0000 at the bottom of the plot change according to the position of the bar.

10.10   Quality print

The plotted data can be displayed in a customised format. To do so the user is expected to click in sub-menu **File** on **Print Preview**.

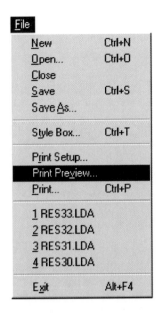

A semi-log graph display will appear which contains all the graphical elements needed for a 'publication quality' plot. The program allows each component of the graph to be chosen at will:

(i)   thickness of x and y axes

(ii)   thickness of the titration line

(iii)   thickness of the confidence limit bar

(iv)   size and kind of the font for the text

(v)   size and kind of the font for the numbers

(vi)   text for y axis (fraction of nonresponding cultures, F_0, or any chosen text)

(vii)   decade labels and tick labels of the y axis

(viii) exponent format of the x axis

(ix)   choice of the x-axis numbering (e.g. every third number shown)

(x)   size and form of the symbols for the experimental points, and whether the symbols are filled or open

(xi)   the log grid on/off

All the above options except (xi) are implemented in **Style Box,** which is to be found in the **File** menu. Switching the grid on and off (xi) is done in the sub-menu **Graph** as shown earlier (p. 159).

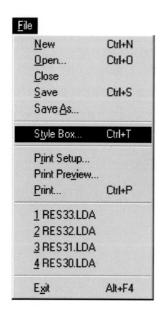

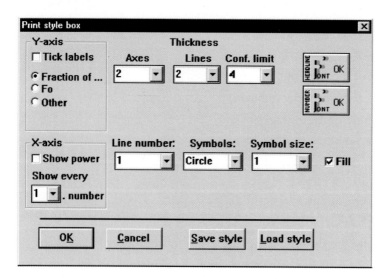

To be able to use a given selection repeatedly, the choices made can be saved by pressing **Save style** . The chosen style can be recalled by clicking on **Load style**.

It is suggested that the reader try various options. A given font size might yield different sizes with different printers, therefore the reader might want to check the variables to achieve a printout which best fits to the project. One should be aware of the fact that in order to obtain a good quality 'black and white' printout the lines of the graph should be black (see comments above). The settings should be saved and used in future experiments.

An example of some of the variables is shown below. Arrows indicate some of the implemented options.

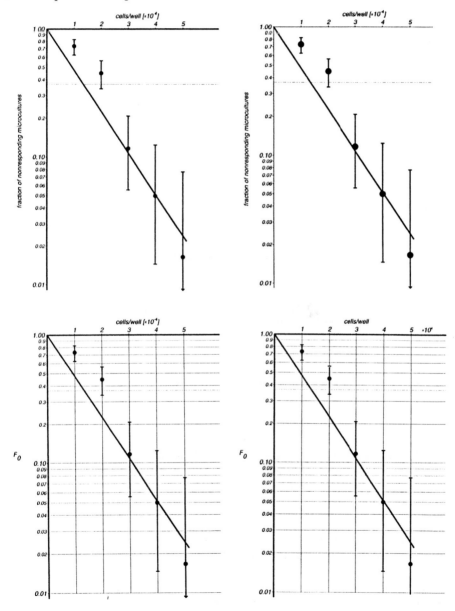

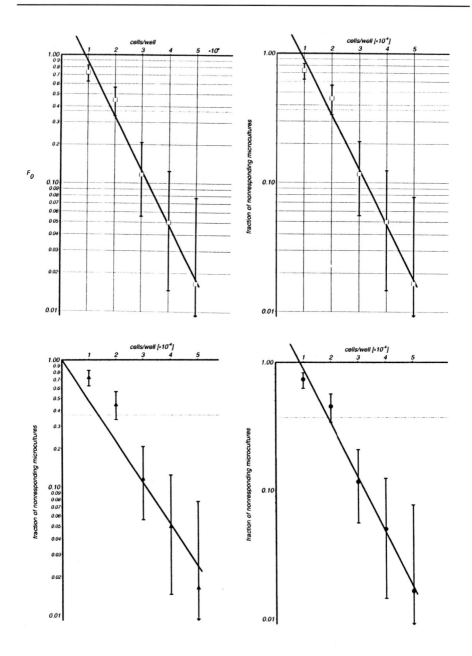

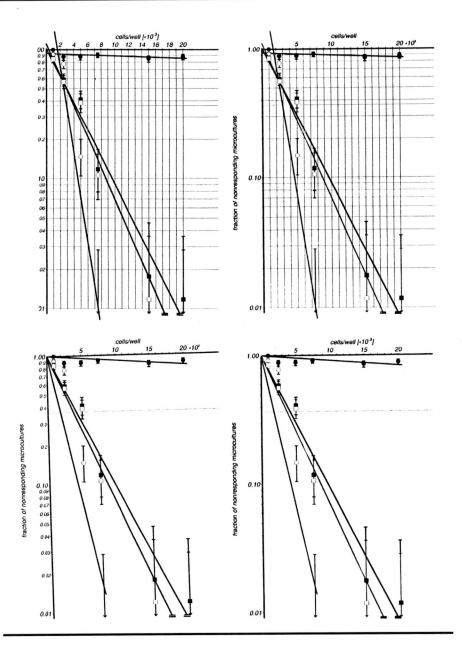

10.11   Summary

This program is satisfactory for most of the tasks encountered in LDA. Beside
the linear regression based on the least square method, there are other models
for fitting a straight line through the experimental points. These include minimal chi-square or maximum likelihood methods. We consider bundling these
options in future versions of the LDA software.

11 Simulation experiments

In the following series of simulation experiments we shall be making use of rectangles and dots, which are intended to represent cultures and cells. In some instances the dots will be red, blue or green, representing cell lineages, namely B, Th or Ts, respectively. Although this chapter is intended to be self-sufficient, it is recommended as companion reading to the LDA program which is an integral part of the book.

The simulation experiments will give the user a sense of what is required to perform a limiting dilution experiment, what kind of results might be obtained and how they can be plotted and interpreted. Since one might in a single session perform a large number of experiments applying many different parameters (e.g. various ratios of T helper cells to B cells) the user will learn what to anticipate in a *real* experiment. Even straightforward repetitions of the same experimental protocol can be useful, since one can come to appreciate the extent to which experimental results can vary due to the Poissonian components.

The 'Simulation program' and the 'LDA program' are two independent software packages, but they have a particularly valuable feature in common which is that they link together. With a click of the mouse – as will be explained towards the end of this chapter – the data from the simulation experiments will be transferred into the LDA program, where they will be processed as if they were real data from a true experiment.

Below we will describe the use of the simulation program step by step.

11.1 Titration of B cells

Upon opening the program a window will appear and the user will be asked to choose from six simulation protocols.

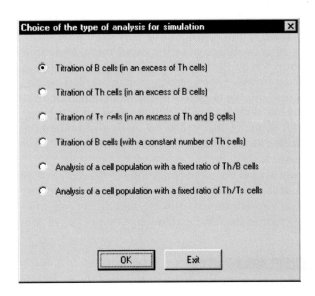

We select **Titration of B cells (in an excess of Th cells)** and click **OK**.

11.1.1 The first decision – are we dealing with rare or abundant cells?

A new window appears with a request to indicate the expected abundance of the cells to be titrated.

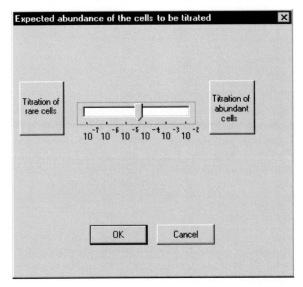

This window realistically reflects one crucial decision-making step. Do we expect to work with cells which are highly abundant or very rare? Obviously, the precise measure of frequency is an objective of the experiment. Nevertheless, in order to get started one has to have a sense of the likely ball-park figure. This crude estimate allows us to choose a *working* range of cell densities, and to estimate total cell numbers, and the numbers of experimental animals to be used. It is clear when working with rare cells that we will need a larger stock cell suspension (thus more animals), than when we analyse abundant cell populations. The computer program will suggest (by default) the cell inputs accordingly.

If we were to choose a highly abundant cell population we would click on the box **Titration of abundant cells**. The other extreme would be to choose **Titration of rare cells**. For our first simulation experiment we will choose a frequency range of about 10^{-3} by moving the tuning arrow to that value. We confirm by clicking **OK**.

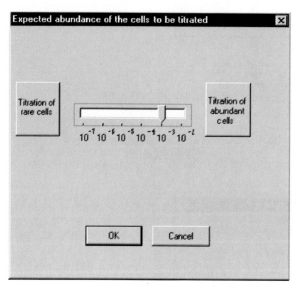

Users should be aware that the simulation program relies on their choice of the frequency only for the purpose of suggesting a series of cell inputs per culture well, and for checking whether there are sufficient cells to perform the experiment. The cell titration that follows this choice is essentially independent of our assessment of abundance.

The titration of B cells has to be performed in an excess of Th cells. We refer to such conditions as 'saturating'. B cells are limiting and Th cells are saturating.

11.1.2 The second decision – how many cells are required, and at what cell density?

In the dialog box **Source of the cells to be titrated** we are prompted to make several rational decisions. We indicate how many cells we intend to make available for the experiment and what the density of the stock cell suspension will be. As a result we will have an estimate of the total volume of the stock cell suspension.

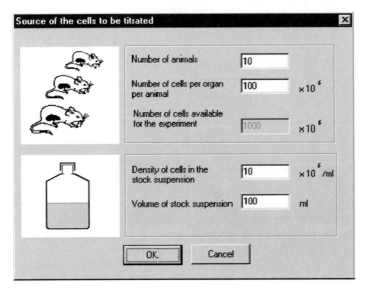

If we perform the experiments at a final cell density of 10^6 cells/ml (from a 10 x stock cell suspension, i.e. 10^7 cells/ml) then with 100 ml cell suspension we will have ample material to carry out most of the experiments. For this particular B cell titration we shall leave the cell requirements at default values (as given in the above window), i.e. we shall work with spleen cells from 10 mice, with a total of 10^9 cells, at the stock cell density of 10^7 cells/ml. Later we shall test what happens if we miscalculate, and have too few cells or an inappropriate cell density.

We confirm by clicking **OK**.

However, if we want to make changes to the previous window (or if we do not remember what we have previously chosen), we can go back to that window by clicking **Cancel** instead of **OK**.

11.1.3 The third decision – the choice of culture system

We have the option to work with Terasaki trays (using 10 µl volumes) or microtitre plates (using 100 µl volumes). We could also choose any other configuration, and we will do so once we get acquainted with the basics.

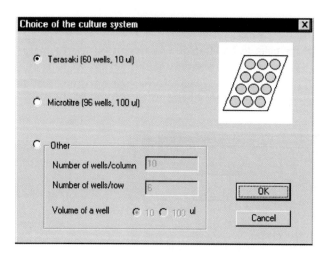

Let us choose the Terasaki system, confirming with **OK**.

11.1.4 The fourth decision – choosing the number of dilutions and cell input/well

Two important decisions have to be made at this point. We will choose the number of dilutions, and also the cell input for each of the dilutions. Maximally, the program allows us to choose six dilutions, and any cell input. Here values of 500, 1000, 2000, 3000, 4000 and 5000 cells/well are suggested by the system.

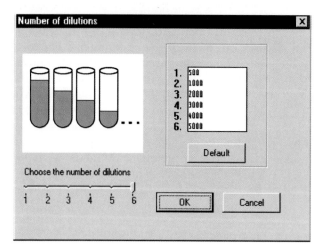

We shall choose five dilutions by shifting the tuning arrow to the left. Changing the number of dilutions from six to five does not simply cut off the highest value (5000 cells/well of the sixth dilution), rather the system proposes a new set of cell inputs. With five dilutions the cell inputs suggested will be 1000, 2000, 3000, 4000 and 5000 cells/well. We could alter any of these. Note that by clicking on **Default** changes of cell input can be reversed to those suggested by the system.

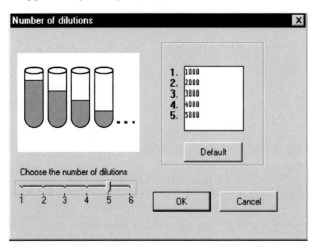

Upon choosing five dilutions and making sure that the default values of cell inputs are displayed, we confirm by clicking **OK**.

11.1.5 Simulation steps

The **LDA – remote 1** box appears and it has several buttons in five rows. Each row stands for one dilution, and each button for an action.

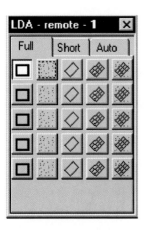

Pressing on the

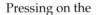 (empty square) indicates that an empty sterile tissue culture container (dish, flask) is available to take up the final volume of 10 ml of the cell suspension

(dots) indicates that one intends to dispense 10 ml of the cell suspension at a given dilution

(rectangle) indicates that one is withdrawing a certain volume of cell suspension (0.6 ml for the Terasaki tray, 9.6 ml for the microtitre plate)

(grid) indicates that one is dispensing the cell suspension into individual wells of the microculture plate followed by a culture period during which the biological process is completed (induction of clonal proliferation, killing, production of cytokines from a single cell or from a clone of cells)

(grid + dots) indicates the readout, that is the assay of positive and negative cultures, or counting and calculating the number of clones in individual microcultures

Before we start the actual simulation let us recapitulate:

- we wish to establish the frequency of B precursor cells in a system in which we assume that the precursor cells are present at a considerably high abundance

- we have sacrificed 10 animals and prepared spleen cell suspension having a total of 1×10^9 cells

- we have chosen to work with 5 dilutions

- we have chosen to use Terasaki trays (60 cultures per dilution, 10 μl/well)

- we have chosen the following cell inputs per microculture

  1000   2000   3000   4000   5000

We are ready to start the simulation.

We assume that the presence of a single B cell in a culture well will give rise to a clone, the antibody product of which is readily detectable. The culture well will score positive even if some or all of the members of the clone eventually die.

Simulation step 1

On the screen, behind the **LDA – remote 1** box, there is a window consisting of two areas:

- a white surface which 'stands for' a sterile tissue culture container (dish, flask), which will be ready to take up the final volume of 10 ml cell suspension

- a red surface onto which data will be written (in other titrations blue and green surfaces will appear)

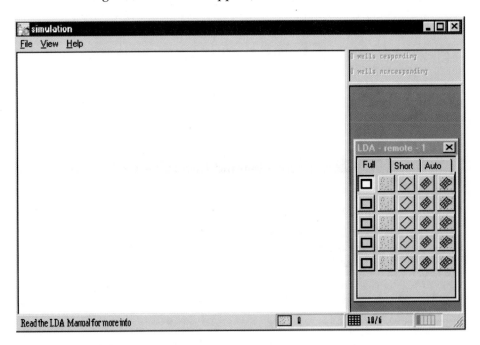

ε bottom there are three icons which signify:

the number of dots present on the white surface (number of precursor cells in the cell suspension)

the culture system chosen (10/6 for Terasaki, 12/8 for microtitre, or any other configuration)

which dilution is being considered (here the first dilution is shown)

For each dilution, when clicking on the button **Empty square**, the empty surface appears. But here, for the first dilution, the empty surface is already on the screen as it appeared simultaneously with the **LDA – remote 1** box. To reiterate, simulation step 1 is the display of an empty surface representing the availability of an empty sterile culture dish ready to receive 10 ml cell suspension.

Simulation step 2

For this particular dilution (dilution 1) we prepare the following cell suspension:

0.1 ml stock cell suspension [10^7/ml]

0.9 ml filler cells* [10^7/ml]

9 ml medium containing antigen and other necessary ingredients*

Total volume 10 ml

Click on the button ▨ (dots), i.e. dispense 10 ml cell mixture. Remember, we chose to work with a frequency of about 10^{-3}. This meant that we dispensed cell numbers estimated to contain the required number of precursor cells. In this example the random number generator positioned 965 dots at random on the white surface (965 precursor cells/culture dish).

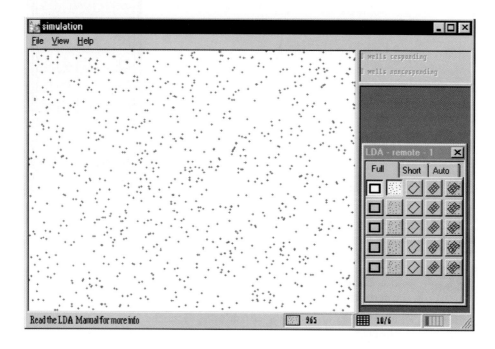

---

* for further details on filler cells and medium composition, antigen and other necessary ingredients see chapter 7. See also the box at the bottom of the next page.

Simulation step 3

Dilution 1 is now ready to be used, i.e. we shall retrieve 0.6 ml (from the total 10 ml) into a pipette or into a dispensing multi-channel instrument.

Click on the button ◇ (rectangle), i.e. draw 0.6 ml into the pipette. A rectangle with an area corresponding to 0.6 ml appears. Since the total area – with all the dots – stood for 10 ml cell suspension, the area of the rectangle covers 6% of the total surface. Note that the position of the rectangle is generated at random (as if you dropped a piece of paper which 'landed' anywhere on the floor).

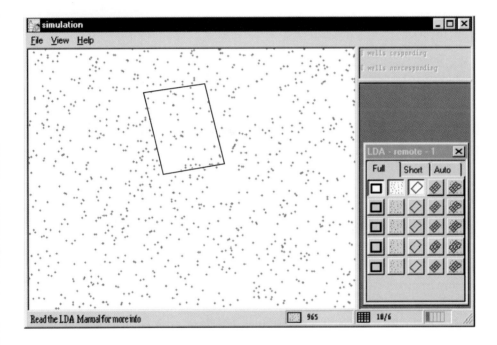

Filler cells do not contribute to the response but keep the requirements for proper culture conditions. Irradiated nude spleen cells make a good source of filler cells. As an alternative one can use Mitomycin C-treated cells or thymus cells. The basic rule is to keep the overall cell density constant.

Simulation step 4

We shall dispense 10 µl aliquots to all 60 wells of the Terasaki tray.

Click on the button [grid icon] (grid) to dispense the cell suspension in 10 µl aliquots to the Terasaki tray

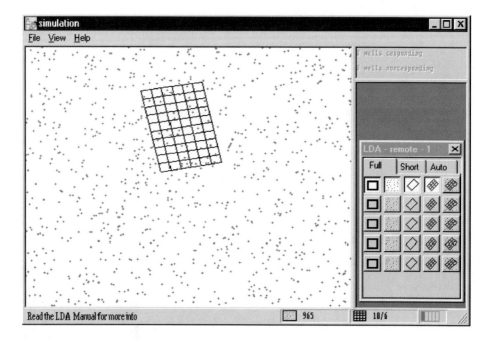

A grid of 6 x 10 squares now covers the area of the Terasaki tray rectangle. Each small square of the grid represents a volume of 10 µl.

The simulation algorithm determines whether a dot is present in an individual small square or not (whether a precursor cell is present in a given microculture or not). At this stage of simulation we shall not yet inspect the grid for the actual presence or absence of dots, for we would not be able to do this in a real experiment.

The Terasaki tray is placed into a humidified CO_2 incubator for an appropriate time interval, say 5 days.

An excess of T help can be achieved by providing an adequate number of T-helper cells, but as an alternative, soluble helper factor can be applied (earlier referred to as 'T-cell replacing factor').

Simulation step 5

Click on the button 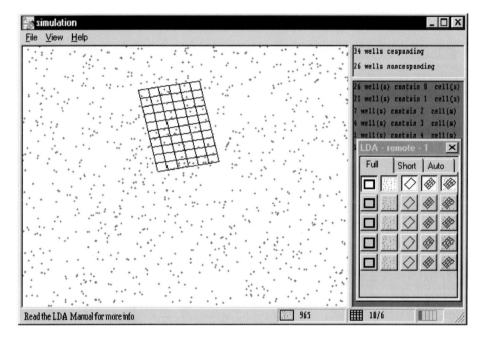 (grid + dots) to retrieve the Terasaki tray from the incubator, and perform a bioassay in order to identify which cultures developed a response. The rule is that those cultures which contain no precursor cells (squares which contain no dots) will be negative, while cultures containing one or more precursor cells (squares with one or more dots) will be positive.

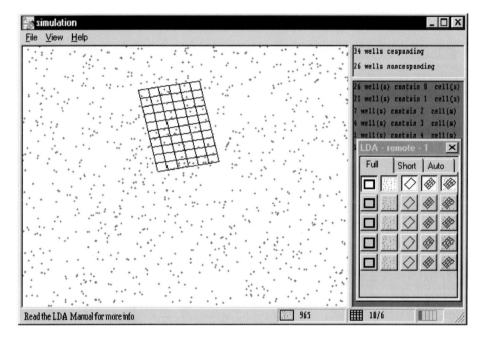

The simulation program provides a detailed account of squares containing given numbers of dots. This particular titration yielded the following results:

26 well(s) contain 0 cells

21 well(s) contain 1 cells

7 well(s) contain 2 cells

4 well(s) contain 3 cells

1 well(s) contain 4 cells

1 well(s) contain 5 cells

These were the results obtained when data were collected for this chapter. The user will obtain similar results, but rarely exactly those given above, since each data set is truly unique and independent of any previously obtained, being newly produced by a random number generator.

From the above detailed account we will only be concerned with the 26 negative and 34 positive cultures. For the moment we shall ignore issues related to multiple clones in individual wells (see Chapter 5), but can move straight on with the next dilution in our simulation experiment.

Simulation step 6

We continue with the next dilution step by clicking on the button 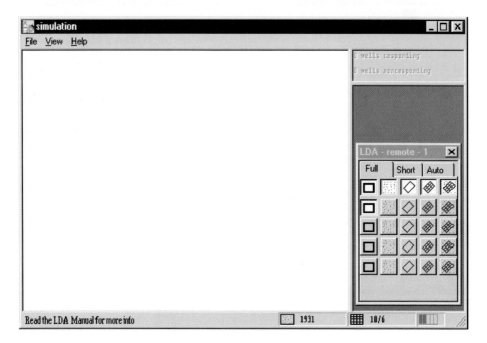 (empty square).

Again a surface will appear which represents the same kind of sterile tissue culture container (dish, flask) as already described in step 1, into which we shall dispense 10 ml cell suspension.

Note that at the bottom of the screen the icon ▐▌ indicates that we are dealing with dilution 2.

Antigen and other necessary ingredients are admixed to the culture media, and the final cell mixture is dispensed into culture wells.

Simulation step 7

For this second dilution we prepare the following cell suspension:

0.2 ml stock cell suspension [10^7 /ml]

0.8 ml filler cells [10^7 /ml]

9 ml medium containing antigen and other necessary ingredients

----

Total volume 10 ml

Click on the button 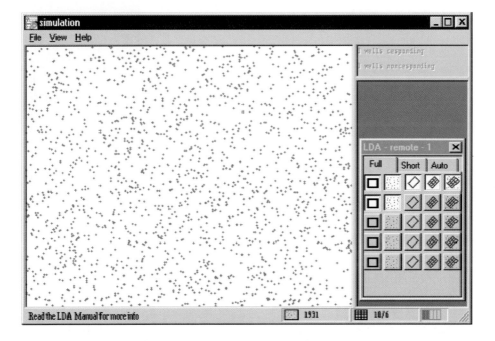 (dots), i.e. dispense 10 ml cell mixture of dilution 2.

The number of cells dispensed will be double that of the first dilution, therefore the number of dots on the white surface area will also be doubled (1931); consequently the number of filler cells added to the mixture will be less, so that the overall cell density will be constant.

> In the past, daily 'feeding' of microcultures was necessary in LDA experiments (1 µl nutritional cocktail was added to each Terasaki well). With an improved medium formula, 'feeding' is often not necessary.

Simulation step 8

From the cell suspension (10 ml of dilution 2) we shall take up 0.6 ml into a pipette or into a dispensing multi-channel instrument.

Click on the button   [◇]   (rectangle), i.e. draw 0.6 ml into the pipette

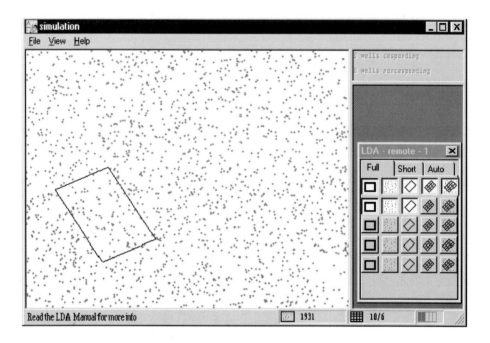

   A rectangle with an area corresponding to 0.6 ml appears. Note that this is positioned differently to the rectangle in step 3. The positioning is *random*, reflecting the process of pipetting, which inevitably retrieves a *random* sample.

Having the correct humidity in the incubator is of utmost importance when using the Terasaki system. Pipetting of sterile saline around the rim of the Terasaki tray, or wrapping the stack of Terasaki trays in Saran foil, helps to minimise evaporation. Microtitre plates are less prone to evaporation problems.

Simulation step 9

We shall dispense 10 μl aliquots into all 60 wells of the Terasaki tray.

Click on the button ⊞ (grid) to dispense the cell suspension in 10 μl aliquots into the Terasaki tray.

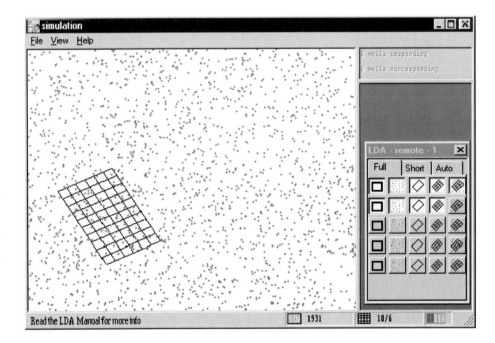

Each of the 60 small squares of the grid represents a volume of 10 μl.

Some squares contain one or more dots, others remain empty. At the stage of distributing the cells into the 10 μl cultures we are not yet able to distinguish those that contain a precursor cell from those that do not, since morphologically all the cells look similar.

The Terasaki tray is placed into a humidified CO_2 incubator for an appropriate time interval, say 5 days.

The simulation provides a detailed account of the number of precursor cells in any given well. In a real experiment we assay either for the soluble product (antibody secreted into the culture media) or for the clonal progeny (the plaque-forming cells).

Simulation step 10

Click on the button 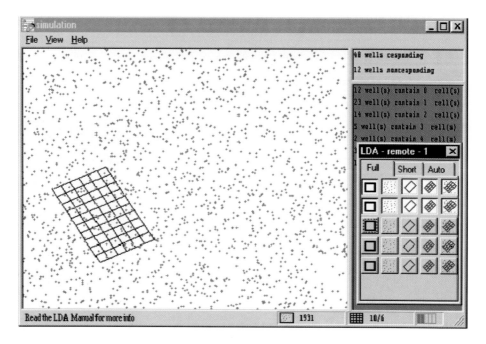 (grid + dots) to retrieve the Terasaki tray from the incubator, and to analyse the response.

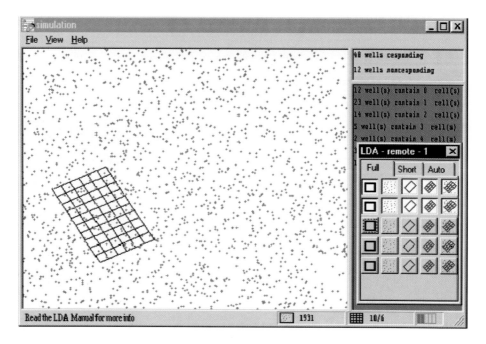

The simulation program provides exact counts for wells containing a given number of dots. Note that rules comparable to those for counting cells in a haemocytometer apply, i.e. cells which 'fall on the grid line' are only counted once.

This particular titration yielded the following results in the 'detailed account':

12 well(s) contain 0 cells

23 well(s) contain 1 cells

14 well(s) contain 2 cells

5 well(s) contain 3 cells

2 well(s) contain 4 cells

3 well(s) contain 5 cells

1 well(s) contain 6 cells

Again, for our purpose, it is sufficient to know that 12 wells were negative and 48 were positive (data on wells containing several cells will be used in another context, also see simulation step 5).

We have described the simulation steps for the first two dilutions. Five buttons were needed for the procedure to run, i.e. from setting up the cultures to performing the assay. For the remaining three dilutions the descriptions are included under:

Simulation steps 11–15 (third dilution)

Simulation steps 16–20 (fourth dilution)

Simulation steps 21–25 (fifth dilution)

Later we shall see that instead of proceeding from button to button, we can perform each dilution in one move. For the reader in a hurry, it may be rewarding to glance at section 11.2.5 before continuing with the simulation.

Simulation steps 11 – 15
Upon clicking the sequence of buttons

Button (empty square)

Button (dots)

Button (rectangle)

Button (grid)

Button (grid + dots)

the set of steps relevant to the third dilution will be executed. Here the composition of the cell suspension will be:

0.3 ml stock cell suspension [10^7 /ml]

0.7 ml filler cells [10^7 /ml]

9 ml medium containing antigen and other necessary ingredients

----

Total volume 10 ml

The final readout of the dots distributed in the Terasaki trays is on the next page.

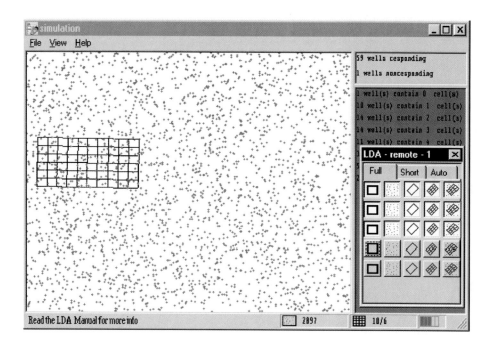

There is 1 negative well and 59 positive ones (the rather complex distribution pattern of cells, e.g. some wells contain 5, 6 or even 7 precursor cells per well [6 and 7 dots / square] is disregarded here).

Simulation steps 16 – 20

Upon clicking the sequence of buttons

Button (empty square)

Button (dots)

Button (rectangle)

Button (grid)

Button (grid + dots)

the simulation steps of the fourth dilution will be executed. The composition of the cell suspension will be:

0.4 ml stock cell suspension [10^7 /ml]

0.6 ml filler cells [10^7 /ml]

9 ml medium containing antigen and other necessary ingredients

----

Total volume 10 ml

The readout of the precursor cell distribution in the Terasaki trays is displayed:

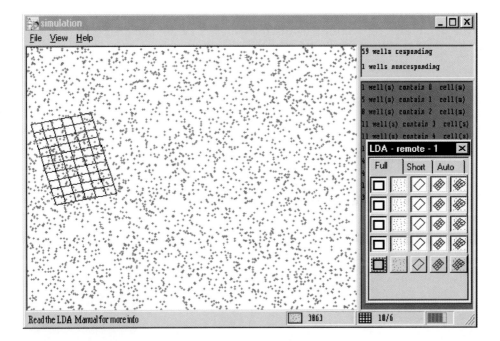

This shows that there was 1 negative well and 59 positive ones (the fact that in the previous dilution and in this one there is the same portion of nonresponding cultures [1/60] should not cause concern. It is part and parcel of the Poisson distribution, as we will see soon when the results are plotted).

If we inspect the distribution of the dots in the window (or still better use a transparent foil with a drawing of the Terasaki grid) we see that the pattern is inhomogenous. This inhomogeneity is a realistic model of the distribution of precursor cells in a cell suspension.

Simulation steps 21 – 25

Upon clicking the sequence of buttons

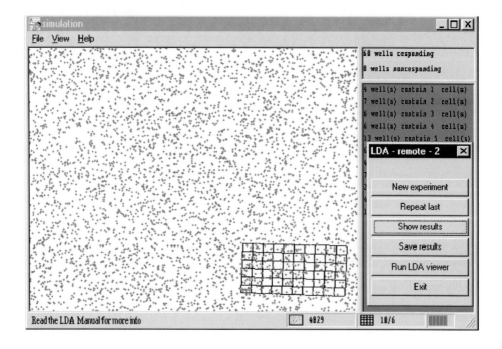

Button (empty square)

Button (dots)

Button (rectangle)

Button (grid)

Button (grid + dots)

the set of steps relevant to the fifth dilution will be executed. Here the composition of the cell suspension will be:

0.5 ml stock cell suspension [10^7 /ml]

0.5 ml filler cells [10^7 /ml]

9 ml medium containing antigen and other necessary ingredients

----

Total volume 10 ml

This shows that no wells were found which lacked a precursor cell. In biological terms all 60 cultures responded (responses in some cultures might have been weaker than in others, but here we follow the response in 'all or none' terms, and the response of a well containing 1 precursor cell is as valid as a response of wells containing 5 precursor cells).

11.1.6 Show results

After all the simulation steps have been completed, the **LDA – remote 2** box appears.

To inspect the results we click on the **Show results** bar. A stack of images of Terasaki trays appears on the screen showing the distribution of precursor cells (red dots) within them.

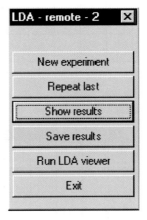

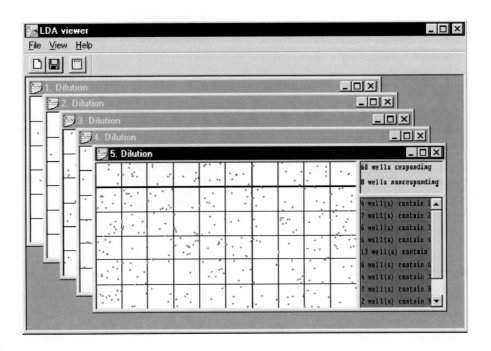

When displayed individually, they look like this:

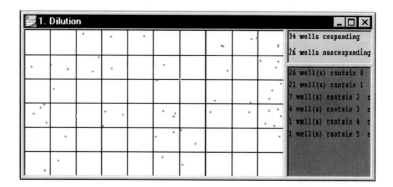

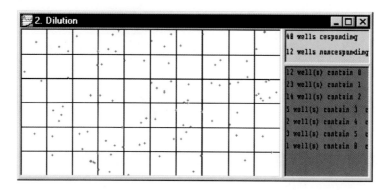

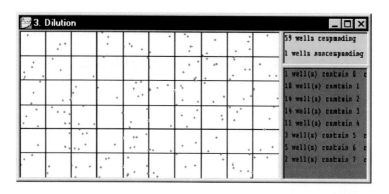

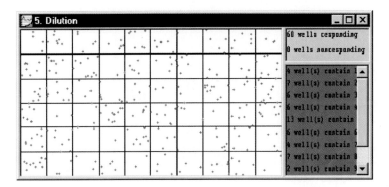

Next to each tray, data on the actual distribution of cells per culture are also given (these will be of some value later when we discuss multi-hit events).

11.1.7 Run LDA viewer

Clicking on **Run LDA viewer** links the simulation program to the actual LDA program. The data from the simulation program become quasi-experimental data on the nonresponding cultures (i.e. containing no precursor cells) and are automatically entered in the table of titrations.

A number of related features of the LDA program are described in Chapter 10 and are also stored under **Help** in the actual program. Briefly, the window is divided into three parts:

- a graph area (semi-log plot)
- a table area (data area, spreadsheet)
- a calculation area (frequencies, confidence limits)

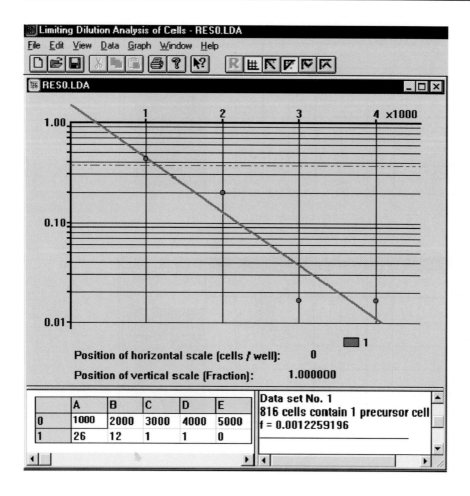

The graph area displays a semi-log plot of the data obtained in the simulation experiment. The straight line is the result of the linear regression calculation based on the points of the simulation experiments. In most instances the regression line does not pass through the origin. This is the case here too. The line intercepts the *x* axis (for the significance of this see Chapter 4). If our assumptions are such that the line should go through the origin (no background, single-hit kinetics – see Chapter 5) we are entitled to force the line through the origin. We shall deal with this issue over the next few pages.

The calculated frequency is displayed in the data area. If the reader finds that the frequency data are not displayed, then clicking on the line **Frequency** in the sub-menu **Graph** provides the calculation.

The frequency data for this experiment show that:

816 cells contain on average 1 precursor cell

$f = 0.001226$

The reader will find it helpful to know the confidence limits, as these provide a range within which the 'true' value of the fraction of nonresponding cultures lies (see section 4.10 and section 3 of the Appendix). To calculate and to display the 95% confidence limits, we click (in the sub-menu **Graph**) first on **Confidence Limits** and thereafter on **Draw Limits**.

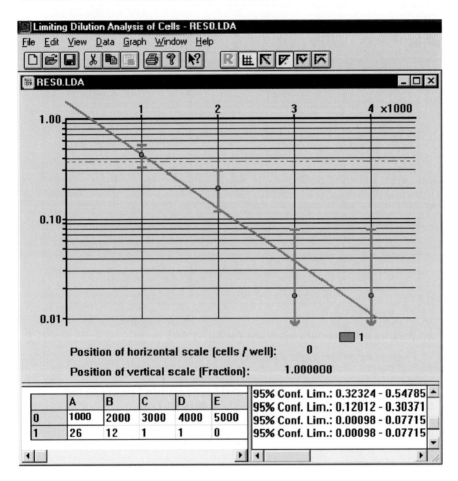

The calculated values of the confidence limits are given in the data area.

As previously mentioned, there are circumstances where the straight line can and should be forced through the origin. For instance, this would be the case when we assume or know that there is no background response, when at the zero input of active cells one can expect all cultures to be nonresponding, and when we are sure that the response conforms to single-hit kinetics. Forcing through the origin is done by selecting **Zero Linear Regression** in the sub-menu

Graph. Clicking on this instantaneously recalculates and replots the new straight line through the origin.

In the same sub-menu **Graph** we can also click on **Frequency**, and this too is calculated and displayed in the lower right area.

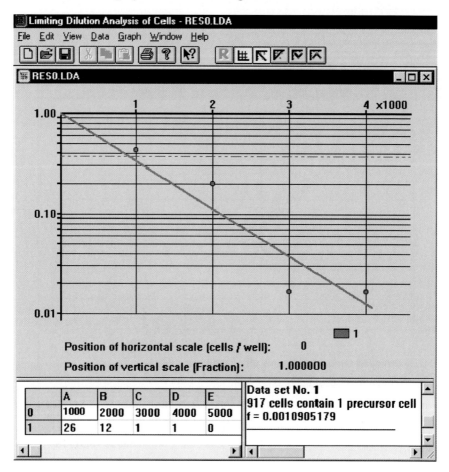

In this particular experiment, where the straight line goes through the origin, the calculation is that:

917 cells contain on average 1 precursor cell

$f = 0.00109$

Again the 95% confidence limits can be displayed, first by selecting **Confidence Limits** in the sub-menu **Graph** and thereafter by clicking on **Draw Limits**.

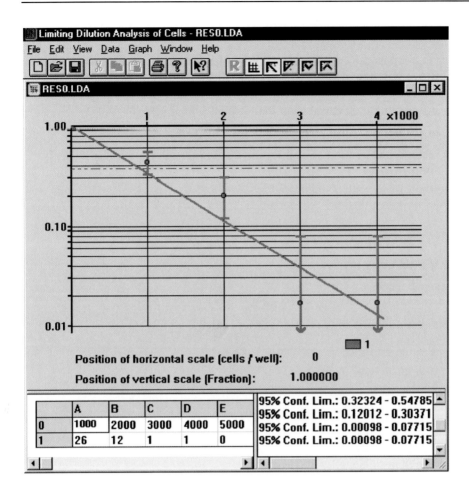

Limiting Dilution Analysis of Cells - RES0.LDA

File Edit View Data Graph Window Help

RES0.LDA

Position of horizontal scale (cells / well): 0

Position of vertical scale (Fraction): 1.000000

	A	B	C	D	E
0	1000	2000	3000	4000	5000
1	26	12	1	1	0

95% Conf. Lim.: 0.32324 - 0.54785
95% Conf. Lim.: 0.12012 - 0.30371
95% Conf. Lim.: 0.00098 - 0.07715
95% Conf. Lim.: 0.00098 - 0.07715

Clearly the 95% confidence limits are identical for both graphical displays, since the limits refer to the experimental points irrespective of whether the line is forced through the origin or not.

The **LDA – remote 2** gives us an opportunity to repeat the experiment. This is done by using newly calculated dot positions obtained by random number generation. The position of the rectangles and the number of nonresponding cultures will vary (in agreement with the Poisson rules). This variation is a feature which the user of this program will come to appreciate on repeated use.

It is suggested that the reader goes through the procedure again at his/her leisure. To do this, click on **Repeat last**. Meanwhile we shall explore modifications of the system.

11.2   B-cell titration – a modification

We shall perform an experiment very similar to the one described in section 11.1 but we will now introduce some modifications. The main changes will be as follows:

- instead of Terasaki trays we shall use microtitre plates
- instead of five dilutions, we shall use only three
- instead of leaving the cell inputs at default values, we shall alter some of them.

We shall work with a spleen cell suspension from 10 mice (1×10^9 cells, 100 ml stock cell suspension, cell density 1×10^7 /ml) as was the case in section 11.1.

11.2.1   First decision step

Titration of B cells

OK

Expected abundance: move tuning arrow to 10^{-3}

OK

11.2.2   Second decision step

All values at default

OK

11.2.3   Third decision step

Microtitre plates (96 wells/ 100 µl each)

OK

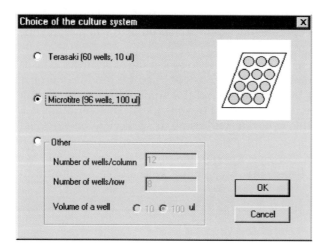

11.2.4 Fourth decision step

Number of dilutions: 3

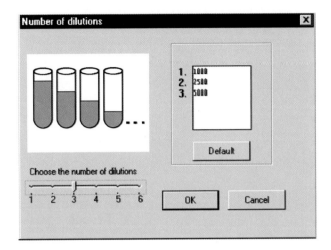

We shall alter the cell input per well: 1000, 3000, 6000

OK

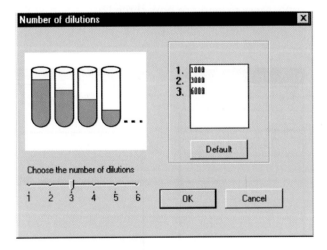

11.2.5 Simulation steps

The **LDA – remote 1** box appears.

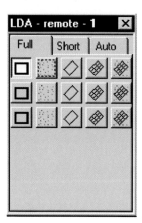

There are now three rows of five buttons active (indicating that we have chosen to perform three dilutions). Instead of engaging each of the fifteen steps, we shall lump them together in rows, such that five steps will be performed in one move. To do this we click on **Short**, upon which the LDA – remote control changes its appearance. There are now three bars, the first of which is active. In three consecutive stages we shall perform all relevant steps of this titration.

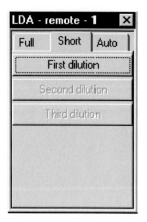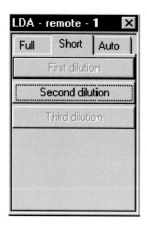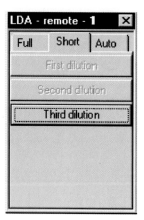

To proceed we must always click on the active bar.

Simulation steps 1 – 5

Upon clicking on [First dilution] all five steps relevant to dilution **one** are performed at once and the results appear on the screen (not shown – summary picture see below).

The five steps are identical to those shown in section 11.1, except that the simulated volumes are different:

step 1: the container for the cell suspension will hold 100 ml (instead of 10 ml of cell suspension used for Terasaki trays).

step 2: 100 ml cell suspension is released into the container

The composition of the cell suspension is:

0.1 ml stock cell suspension [10^7 /ml]

9.9 ml filler cells [10^7 /ml]

90 ml medium containing antigen and other necessary ingredients

----

Total volume 100 ml

----

step 3: 9.6 ml of the cell suspension is retrieved into a pipette or into a multi-channel instrument (instead of 0.6 ml for Terasaki trays)

step 4: 100 ml aliquots are released into the microtitre plates (instead of 10 ml for Terasaki trays) and these are placed into an incubator for 5 days

step 5: the culture trays are retrieved from the incubator, and by bioassay the number of responding cultures is established

Simulation steps 6 – 10

We click on [Second dilution] to simulate the steps relevant to the **second** dilution

step 6: the container for pipetting 100 ml cell suspension is prepared

step 7: 100 ml cell suspension is released into the container

The composition of the cell suspension is:

0.3 ml stock cell suspension [10^7 /ml]

9.7 ml filler cells [10^7 /ml]

90 ml medium containing antigen and other necessary ingredients

----

Total volume 100 ml

----

step 8: 9.6 ml of the cell suspension is retrieved into a pipette or into a multi-channel instrument

step 9: 100 ml aliquots are released into the microtitre plates and these are placed into an incubator for 5 days

step 10: the culture trays are retrieved from the incubator, and by bioassay the number of responding cultures is established

Simulation steps 11 – 15

We click on [Third dilution] to simulate the steps relevant to the **third** dilution

step 11: the container for pipetting 100 ml cell suspension is prepared

step 12: 100 ml cell suspension is released into the container

The composition of the cell suspension is:

0.6 ml stock cell suspension [10^7 /ml]

9.4 ml filler cells [10^7 /ml]

90 ml medium containing antigen and other necessary ingredients

----

Total volume 100 ml

----

step 13: 9.6 ml of the cell suspension is retrieved into a pipette or into a multi-channel instrument

step 14: 100 µl aliquots are released into the microtitre plates and these are placed into an incubator for 5 days

step 15: the culture trays are retrieved from the incubator, and by bioassay the number of responding cultures is established

Note that in most of the experiments we use a vast excess of filler cells; these cells serve to maintain a constant cell density. In the simulation experiments we have chosen 10^7 /ml as final cell density. If we performed titrations in which the expected frequency of precursor cells were 10 times or even 100 times lower, proportionally more titrated cells would be used as 'input/well' and fewer filler cells would be required to compensate the cell density (see Chapters 5 and 7).

11.2.6 *Show results*

After consecutively clicking on all three bars, the **LDA – remote 2** box appears.

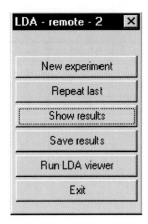

We click on the 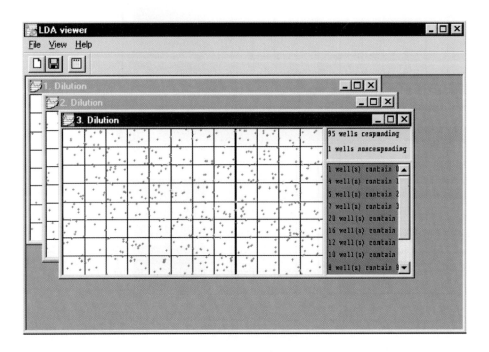 bar and a stack of three images of microtitre plates appears on the screen, showing the distribution of cells (red dots) within them.

When displayed individually they look like this

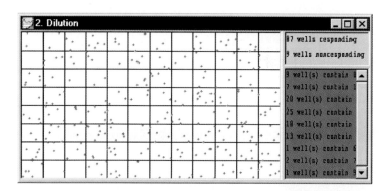

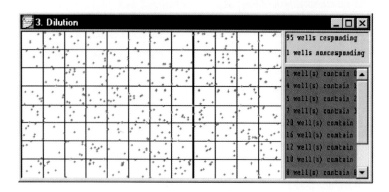

Data on the actual distribution of precursor cells per well are given next to each tray. They will be disregarded in the ensuing exercise.

11.2.7 Run LDA viewer

Click on ┃ Run LDA viewer ┃ and the semi-log plot appears.

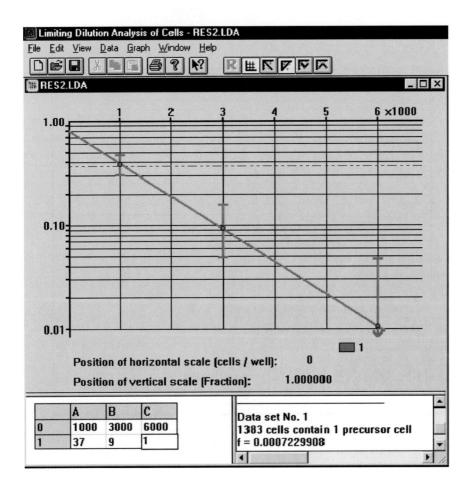

95% confidence limits will be displayed by selecting **Confidence Limits** in the sub-menu **Graph** and thereafter by clicking on **Draw Limits**. We calculate the frequency by choosing **Frequency** in the same sub-menu, **Graph** .

The calculated frequency (as displayed in the data area) is:

1383 cells contain on average 1 precursor cell

$f = 0.000723$

The straight line can be forced to go through the origin. This is achieved by choosing **Zero Linear Regression** in the sub-menu **Graph**. The calculations are performed by clicking on **Frequency** in the same sub-menu **Graph** (displayed in the data area; to inspect all data be sure to scroll through completely).

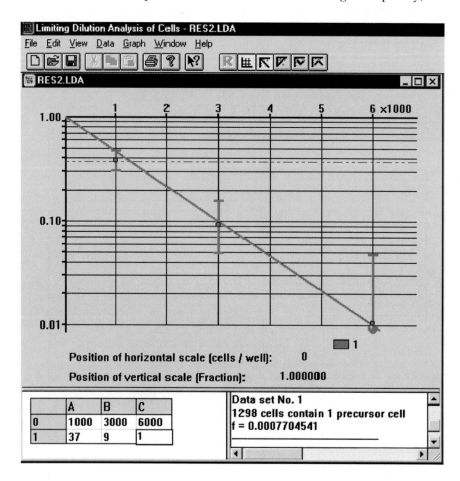

In the next section we shall consider other titrations.

When clicking on **Graph** the format of the semi-log plot changes. The log grid can be switched on and off, the regression line can be drawn or the experimental points can be connected.

11.3   Titration of Th cells

We shall simulate the titration of Th-precursor cells in exactly the same manner as already described for B cells (sections 11.1 and 11.2), except that now the dots are blue instead of red. This exercise is useful precisely because it is similar – it is a preparatory step for simulations which involve two or more cell populations. Note that it is to be assumed that the cells which are limiting in the culture system are the Th-precursor cells, while B-precursor cells are present in excess. In practical terms this means that while each well contains several B-precursor cells, it may or may not contain a Th-precursor cell. B cells will not respond in the absence of Th cells.

We choose   ⌀   Titration of Th cells (in an excess of B cells)

11.3.1 First decision step
Expected abundance: move tuning arrow to 10^{-5}

11.3.2 Second decision step
We leave all values at default, i.e.
- 10 animals
- 10^8 cells/spleen
- 10^7 cells/ml
- 100 ml cell suspension

11.3.3 Third decision step
We choose microtitre plates (96 wells, 100 μl each)

11.3.4 Fourth decision step
We choose 6 dilutions and leave the default values for the cell input

$$5 \times 10^4, \quad 10 \times 10^4, \quad 20 \times 10^4, \quad 30 \times 10^4, \quad 40 \times 10^4, \quad 50 \times 10^4$$

Be aware that the above cell inputs are correct when using microtitre plates. If we were to try and use the Terasaki system, the program would point out that the chosen cell density (10^7 cells/ml) is too low for the planned titration to be performed. A warning appears on the screen, and we are informed that we have to work with a higher (stock) cell density or, alternatively, use larger culture wells. As the wells of the microtitre system are ten-fold larger, our chosen cell density is adequate.

11.3.5 Simulation steps

We have chosen to work with a considerably higher cell input than we did in sections 11.1 or 11.2: there it did not matter if we prepared 10 ml or 100 ml cell suspension (apart from the cost of the medium). With inputs of the magnitude of 10^4 cells/well or higher, we would probably prepare *just enough* cell suspension to fill the required number of culture trays. Obviously we would not prepare dilutions in volumes of 100 ml if we intended to use just about 10 ml.

Contrary to real experimentation, here in the simulation we shall continue to work *wastefully*, as the simulation surface has to be manifoldly larger than the final grid, otherwise we could not ensure and visualise a genuine random sampling.

Although the simulation surface assumes a cell suspension volume of 100 ml, in Table 11.1 the titration protocol for a final volume of 10 ml (sufficient to fill one microtitre plate) is given.

Table 11.1. Titration protocol

Dilution	Stock T cell suspension (ml)	Filler cells (ml)	B cells + ingredients (ag, etc.) (ml)
1st	0.5	4.5	5
2nd	1	4	5
3rd	2	3	5
4th	3	2	5
5th	4	1	5
6th	5		5
Total	15.5	14.5	30

Simulation volumes are 10 times higher, as explained in this text.

Note that whenever we use larger volumes than chosen at the outset, a warning window alerts us to this: as in the case here, since the simulation requires 155 ml (5 + 10 + 20 + 30 + 40 + 50 ml) cell suspension. Nevertheless, we are allowed to continue with the simulation despite the warning. Incidentally, although the procedure allows us now to disregard the suggested amount of cell suspension, it would prevent us from continuing if the cell density of the stock suspension were lower than the final density in the culture. In this experiment we do not encounter this obstacle.

We choose the *short* version by enabling **Short** on the **LDA – remote 1** box and then we click the 1st, 2nd ... 6th dilution bars, consecutively. The simulated results in the 8 x 12 grid indicate the outcome for each of the chosen dilutions.

11.3.6 *Show results*

After clicking consecutively on all six bars, the **LDA – remote 2** box appears. We click on the **Show results** bar and a stack of six images of microtitre plates appears which show the distribution of Th-precursor cells (blue dots) within them:

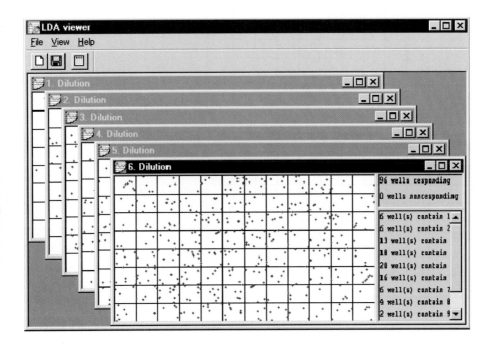

The following two pages show how the images look when spread out separately.

The program settings prevent us from continuing the simulation if the cell density chosen for the stock cell suspension is lower than the final cell density of the culture.

The 'Show results' step is not obligatory: instead, the 'Run LDA viewer' can be pressed to view the results as a semi-log plot.

1. Dilution

37 wells responding
59 wells nonresponding

59 well(s) contain 0
31 well(s) contain 1
4 well(s) contain 2 c
2 well(s) contain 3 c

2. Dilution

52 wells responding
44 wells nonresponding

44 well(s) contain 0
31 well(s) contain 1
13 well(s) contain 2
7 well(s) contain 3 c
1 well(s) contain 4 c

3. Dilution

84 wells responding
12 wells nonresponding

12 well(s) contain 0
24 well(s) contain 1
29 well(s) contain 2
19 well(s) contain 3
5 well(s) contain 4 c
3 well(s) contain 5 c
4 well(s) contain 6 c

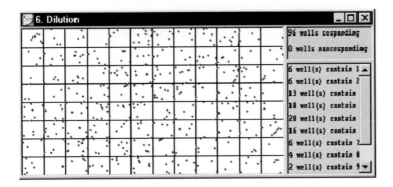

Data on the actual distribution of cells per well are given next to each micro-titre plate, but they can be disregarded here.

11.3.7 *Run LDA viewer*

Click on | Run LDA viewer | and a semi-log plot appears. Choosing **Frequency** in the sub-menu **Graph** performs the calculation of the frequency which is displayed in the data area:

113 335 cells contain on average 1 precursor cell

$f = 0.0000088234$

We can now calculate and display the 95% confidence limits:

(Graph   Confidence Limits   Draw Limits)

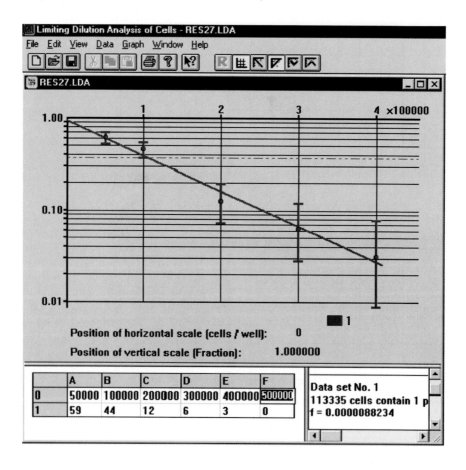

This plot displays the standard linear regression line. It happens to closely resemble the plot with the regression line forced through the origin. To compare the two lines click on:

(**Graph   No Zero Linear Regression**)

(**Graph   Zero Linear Regression**)

It is useful to connect the experimental points:

(**Graph   Connect Points**)

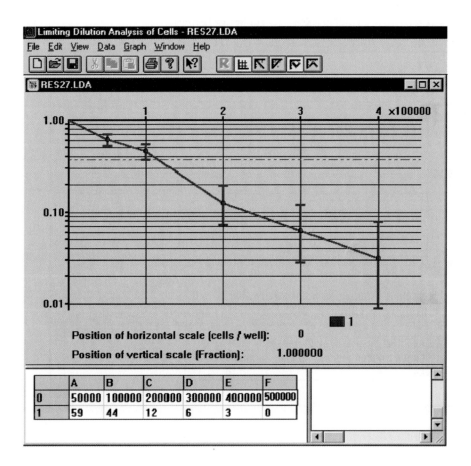

Other features of the semi-log plot are explained in Chapter 10 where the LDA program is described.

We now wish to address an important point. The plot only displays data from those dilutions where *not* all cultures respond. In this experiment the highest input (500 000 cells/well) is disregarded because here all cultures responded. If we wish to establish how the titration looks if say one culture were negative, then we would choose **Consider 0 as 1** in sub-menu **Graph**. This does not alter the tabulated data (zero remains zero) but it changes the plot instantaneously, where six experimental points are now plotted instead of five. This option can be very useful in simulation experiments as well as in actual LDA experiments.

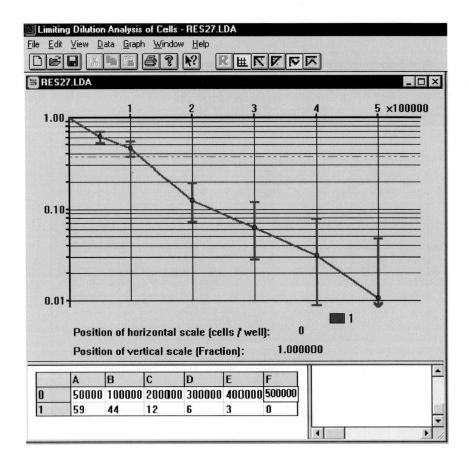

In this plot, the options **Zero Linear Regression, No Zero Linear Regression** and **Connect Points** can be dealt with in the same way as shown in the previous examples.

> When the plot is based on 'Connect Points', rather than 'Linear regression', *Frequency calculation* is disabled.

11.4   Titration of Ts cells

To simulate the titration of suppressor cells (any inhibitory or downregulating cell) we use a similar set of assumptions as we used for B cells and Th cells. The final readout will be different: those wells which lack a suppressor cell will respond. Clearly there are some suppressor cell assays in which the presence of a suppressor cell leads to a 'positive signal' (e.g. chromium release in cytotoxic tests). In this simulation experiment, the suppressor cell is a model for all instances when the 'signal is extinguished'.

We choose ○ Titration of Ts cells (in an excess of Th and B cells)

11.4.1 First decision step

Expected abundance: move tuning arrow to 10^{-5}

11.4.2 Second decision step

We leave all values at default, i.e.

- 10 animals
- 10^8 cells/spleen
- 10^7 cells/ml
- 100 ml cell suspension

11.4.3 Third decision step

We choose microtitre plates (96 wells, 100 µl each)

11.4.4 Fourth decision step

We choose 2 dilutions and leave the default values for the cell input

1×10^5, 3×10^5

11.4.5 Simulation steps

The composition of the cell suspension is listed below.

Table 11.2. Titration protocol (all cell suspensions at 10^7/ml)

Dilution	Stock Ts cell suspension (ml)	Filler cells (ml)	Th cells (ml)	B cells + ingredients (ag, etc.) (ml)
1st	1	2	2	5
2nd	3		2	5

Here the total volume is 10 ml which is sufficient to fill one microtitre plate. The sampling procedure of the simulation program assumes a ten-fold excess of the cell suspension.

We choose the *short* version by enabling **Short** on **LDA – remote 1** and then we click on the 1st and 2nd dilution bars consecutively. The simulated results in the 8 x 12 grid indicate the outcome for the chosen dilutions. Be aware that in the green area, data are given on the number of wells which contain 0, 1, 2, 3 .... suppressor cells. Wells containing a Ts cell will not respond (*only the negative cultures are positive*). A summary of the results will be obtained upon completion of the next step.

11.4.6 Show results

We click on [**Show results**]

Two stacked images of microtitre plates appear. When laid out separately they look like this:

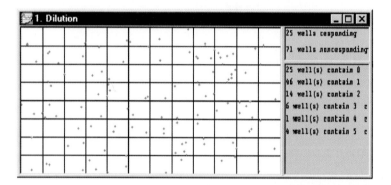

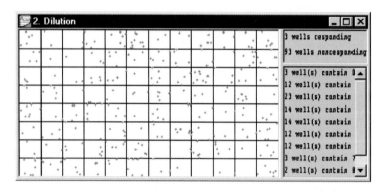

Data on the actual distribution of cells per well are given next to each tray. Once again, only wells which do not contain a suppressor cell respond.

11.4.7 *Run LDA viewer*

We click on Run LDA viewer and the semi-log plot appears:

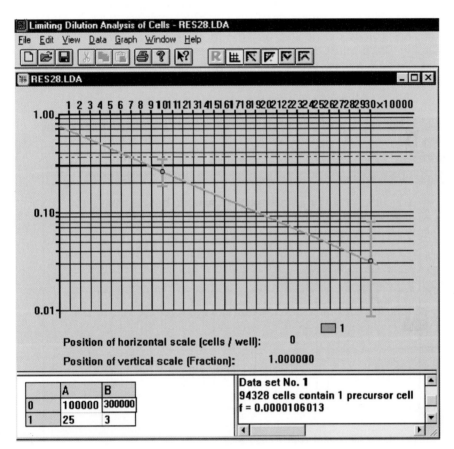

Now that we are ready to do the frequency calculations and to establish the 95% confidence limits, we should be aware of the fact that the data in the table (lower left) show the number of responding wells (rather than nonresponding ones, as was the case in all previous experiments). These responding wells are considered as the basis for the calculation of the zero term of the Poisson distribution.

Choosing **Frequency** in the sub-menu **Graph** performs the calculation of the frequency which is displayed in the data area:

94328 cells contain on average 1 precursor cell

$f = 0.0000106$

After displaying 95% confidence limits (**Confidence Limits, Draw Limits**) we shall also show a plot based on connecting experimental points. We shall do this by presenting the fraction of cultures which *do* contain suppressor cells. We choose **Settings** in the sub-menu **Graph** and activate the line m responding (be aware that for the analysis of suppressor cells, or any cells which have an 'inhibitory property', the definitions of responding and nonresponding cultures are exactly the reverse of those in all previous examples). Now we shall apply **Graph** and **Connect Points without zero.**

It would be wrong to connect points to the origin since this would imply that with *no* input of suppressor cells the cultures *do not* respond – in fact they do.

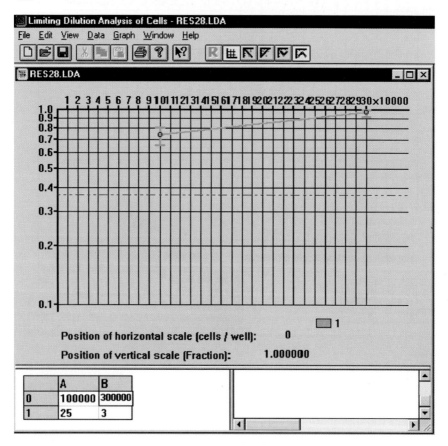

11.5 Titration of B cells with a constant number of Th cells

As in previous titrations, here we shall also titrate *one* cell population (B cells), but we shall introduce an additional parameter which is that the supply of the Th cells (required for the response) is restricted.

We choose   ○   Titration of B cells (with a constant number of Th cells)

and click OK. The dialogue box '**Titrations...**' appears

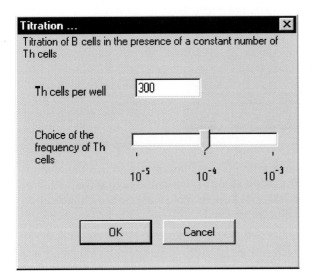

    Decisions on two parameters are required: (i) how many Th cells do we intend to distribute into each microculture well, and (ii) what is the frequency of Th-precursor cells among these cells? Some background knowledge is required to perform this simulation experiment and so the reader is referred to sections 5.5, 5.7 and 7.4. Briefly, we want to know what happens if we perform a B-cell titration with *inadequate numbers* of Th cells (in contrast to the results obtained under conditions of Th-cell saturation, which were already seen in section 11.3).

> Limiting dilution experiments sometimes yield a 'stagnating' response. This 'levelling off' signifies that the number of cells required to support the response of the titrated cells is inadequate.

We choose a modest input of 1000 Th cells per well and move the tuning arrow to a value of about 8×10^{-4} (i.e. almost $1/1000$).

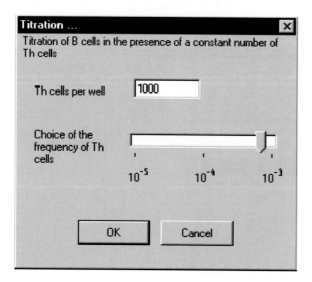

We should be aware of the fact that both in a simulation and in a real experiment, we make a decision on the Th-cell input, while the actual frequency of Th cells in this population is usually not known. We shall test how the titration is affected by variations in Th-cell frequency.

All the remaining steps of the simulation are performed as they were described in the previous sections. Thus:

11.5.1 *First decision step*

Expected abundance: move tuning arrow to 10^{-5}

11.5.2 *Second decision step*

We leave all values at default, i.e.

- 10 animals
- 10^8 cells/spleen
- 10^7 cells/ml
- 100 ml cell suspension

11.5.3 *Third decision step*

We choose microtitre plates (96 wells, 100 µl each)

11.5.4 Fourth decision step

We choose 6 dilutions and leave the default values for the cell input

$$5 \times 10^4, \quad 10 \times 10^4, \quad 20 \times 10^4, \quad 30 \times 10^4, \quad 40 \times 10^4, \quad 50 \times 10^4$$

11.5.5 Simulation steps

The composition of the cell suspension is listed below; it is given for a volume of 10 ml which is sufficient to fill one microtitre plate.

Table 11.3. Titration protocol

Dilution	Stock B cell suspension (ml)	Irradiated B cells (ml)	T cells + ingredients (ag, etc.) (ml)
1st	0.5	4.5	5
2nd	1	4	5
3rd	2	3	5
4th	3	2	5
5th	4	1	5
6th	5		5

The simulation surface assumes a cell suspension volume of 100 ml from which 9.6 ml is sampled. Thus the volume of the cell suspension used is 10 times larger than needed.

The relative proportion of all components is the same in both tables. We are just more *wasteful* so as to be correct about the Poissonian sampling (note that whenever we use larger volumes of cell suspension than we indicated at the outset of the simulation, a warning window will alert us; the experiment can be continued in spite of this warning – just click **OK**).

By clicking on the 1st, 2nd ... 6th dilution bars on the **LDA – remote 1** (**Short**) consecutively, we obtain the simulation of the Poisson distribution of B cells (red dots) and of T cells (blue dots). In previous simulations, the data area was red *or* blue, here both colours are used. Move the separator to view the entire width of the data area. Productive combinations, i.e. the number of wells containing one or more B *and* Th-precursor cells, are indicated on the white area.

'Levelling off' often remains unnoticed especially when too few dilutions and only a small number of cultures are used.

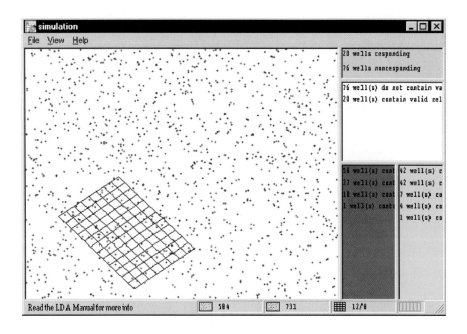

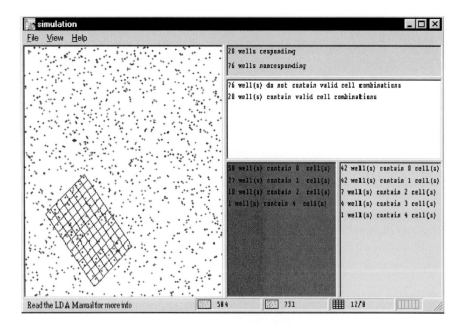

'Levelling off' may also be mistaken for inhibition.

11.5.6 *Show results*

Clicking on **Show results (LDA – remote 2)** displays the stack of 6 images of microtitre plates which show the distribution of B- and Th-precursor cells (red and blue dots).

As we went through this step in detail in previous dilutions we will only display the first dilution.

Moving the line separator increases the data area:

In the area with the red background F_0, F_1, F_2 ... terms of B-cell distribution are given, while on the blue background F_0, F_1, F_2 ... terms of Th distribution are shown. In the white area the productive combinations (at least one B-cell precursor and one T-cell precursor) are displayed.

11.5.7 Run LDA viewer

Click on | Run LDA viewer | and a semi-log plot appears.

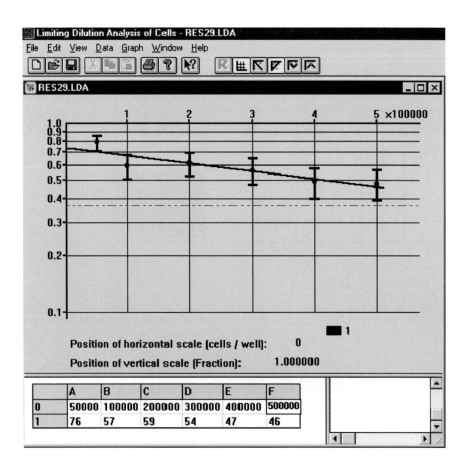

The reader should realise that since we supply the Th cells in 'frugal' quantities, the titration will not adhere to single-hit kinetics. In fact the response will 'level off' (see section 5.7). If we pretended not to know this (in real experimentation this might be true) we could still draw the regression line and calculate the frequency. But the correct way to use the data is to connect points (from the sub-menu **Graph** we choose **Connect Points**).

When 'levelling off' is suspected, drawing linear regression lines and the subsequent calculation of frequencies should be avoided.

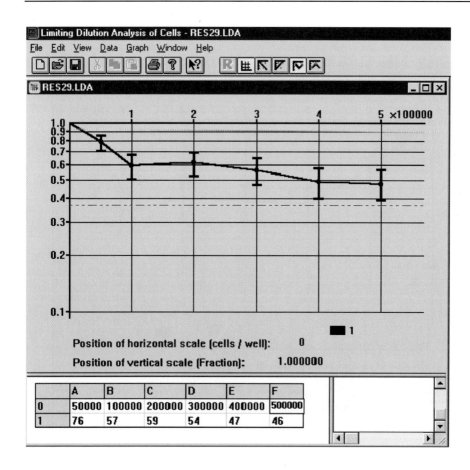

We shall return to this titration in section 11.8 when we deal with chi-square calculations.

We do not calculate the frequency (incidentally, when the **Connect Points** option is used, the frequency calculation is disabled [grey]). The reader is encouraged to perform this experiment keeping all the values the same, but adding 3000 Th cells/well (instead of 1000). The final plot (using **Connect Points**) is given on the next page.

When the 'Connect Points' option is used, the frequency calculation is disabled. The points are usually connected to origin, except with a titration of Ts cells when this is not permitted.

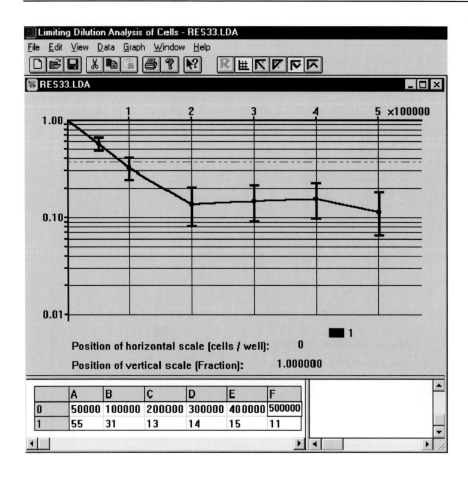

Although we have refrained from going into too much detail on the theoretical implications, the reader should have noticed that one and the same titration of B cells leads to profoundly different results depending on the number of Th cells added (compare the last two figures). The take-home lesson from this experiment is that it is of utmost importance to work with an excess of all components, while limiting only the titrated component (this is true providing that the excess of one given component is not deleterious to another).

11.6 Analysis of a cell population with a fixed ratio of Th/B cells

This is a somewhat different simulation. We avoid calling it 'titration', since we analyse the effect of diluting two components simultaneously. Assuming that by now readers are fully acquainted with the procedures described in earlier pages, we shall no longer hold them by the hand and we shall only explain those steps which differ from previous ones.

We choose   ○ Analysis of a cell population with a fixed ratio of Th/B cells

The only window differing from the previous set is the following:

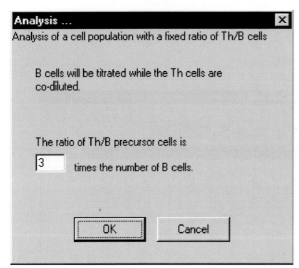

Let us assume that the cell suspension is composed of a three-fold excess of Th-precursor cells. The other parameters differ only slightly from those of section 11.5.

11.6.1 *First decision step*

Expected abundance: move tuning arrow to 3×10^{-5}

11.6.2 *Second decision step*

We leave all values at default, i.e.

- 10 animals
- 10^8 cells/spleen
- 10^7 cells/ml
- 100 ml cell suspension

11.6.3 *Third decision step*

We choose microtitre plates (96 wells, 100 μl each)

11.6.4 *Fourth decision step*

We choose 6 dilutions and leave the default values for the cell input

$$1 \times 10^4, \quad 25 \times 10^4, \quad 5 \times 10^4, \quad 10 \times 10^4, \quad 15 \times 10^4, \quad 20 \times 10^4$$

11.6.5 *Simulation steps*

LDA – remote 1 *short*; 1st to 6th dilution

11.6.6 *Show results*

LDA – remote 2; Show results

11.6.7 *Run LDA viewer*

A semi-log plot appears (leave the option of linear regression not going through the origin). Frequency calculation reveals: 30 880 cells contain on average 1 precursor cell; $f = 0.000324$

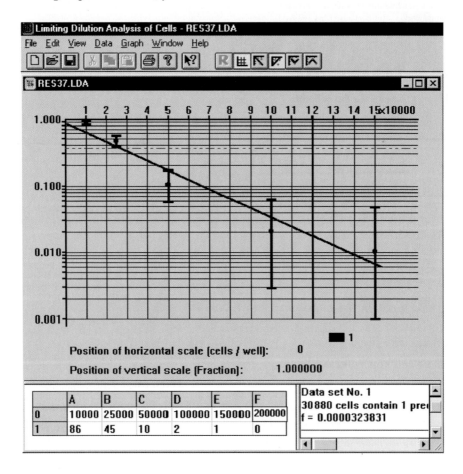

A similar titration with a **Connect Points** display is shown below:

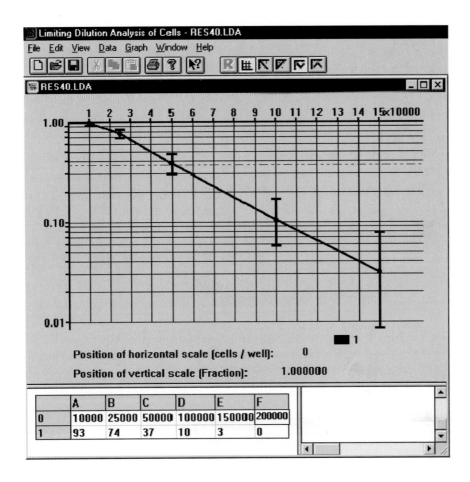

The reader is advised to repeat the simulation but with an altered proportion of Th cells to B cells. We can perform this in a range of 0.1 x to 10 x. (Higher or lower values are disabled by the system.)

We should be aware of the fact that B-cell titration in the presence of a low multiplicity of Th cells cannot give an accurate measure of the B-cell frequency. Rather, it reflects the rarer population, i.e. the frequency of Th cells. The take-home lesson is that we should always ascertain that the titration which we perform reflects the cell population which we intend to titrate. For further interpretation the reader is advised to refer to Chapter 5 on multi-target events.

11.7   Analysis of a cell population with a fixed ratio of Th/Ts cells

The analysis of the mixture of Th/Ts cells follows the same rules as described above (section 11.6), though the plotted results will be very different. The Ts cells have a *model* function; they represent cells which have an inhibitory, suppressive or killing property. We assume that the presence of such a cell will prevent a response from taking place. Before embarking on the Th/Ts analysis, the user should read sections 6.1 and 7.5, and bear in mind the following three rules:

- cultures not containing a Th-precursor cell will be negative
- cultures containing a Th-precursor cell (in absence of Ts) will be positive
- cultures containing a Ts precursor cell will be negative

(it is a B-cell response; Ts cells eliminate Th function but do not abrogate B-cell function).

Again we assume that the reader has already mastered the simulation procedure, and so we shall indicate only those steps which differ from the previous titration.

We choose   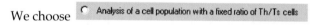 Analysis of a cell population with a fixed ratio of Th/Ts cells

Let us assume that we are dealing with a cell suspension which has a 1 : 1 ratio of Th : Ts precursor cells. In the next window we select '1'. **The ratio of Th/Ts precursor cells is such that there is a 1 fold excess of Ts cells** (ungrammatical for '1', but correct for higher numbers, e.g. '3').

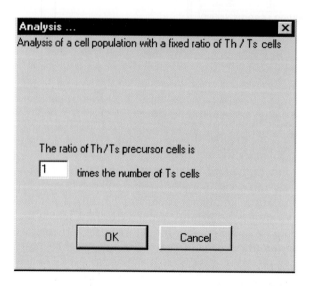

11.7.1 First decision step

Expected abundance: move tuning arrow to 3×10^{-5}

11.7.2 Second decision step

We leave all values at default, i.e.

- 10 animals
- 10^8 cells/spleen
- 10^7 cells/ml
- 100 ml cell suspension

11.7.3 Third decision step

We choose microtitre plates (96 wells, 100 μl each)

11.7.4 Fourth decision step

We choose 6 dilutions and leave the default values for the cell input

$$1 \times 10^4, \quad 25 \times 10^4, \quad 5 \times 10^4, \quad 10 \times 10^4, \quad 15 \times 10^4, 20 \times 10^4$$

11.7.5 Simulation steps

LDA – remote 1; Short ; 1st to 6th dilution

11.7.6 Show results

LDA – remote 2; Show results

11.7.7 Run LDA viewer

A semi-log plot appears (alter the option of linear regression to **Connect Points**).

The titration shows a bimodal shape – help and inhibition. Note that here it is right to connect points to the origin (see also section 11.3), since at zero input of Th + Ts cells cultures contain B cells but yield no response. At a low input of titrated cells, helper cells are present in some wells, while rare Ts cells are present in others. Only at a higher input do Ts cells interfere with T-helper activity.

Suspected 'levelling off' can be visualised by performing one full-range titration (so that the cultures are supplemented with chosen 'saturating' cell populations) in parallel with another titration where we double the 'saturating' cell population.

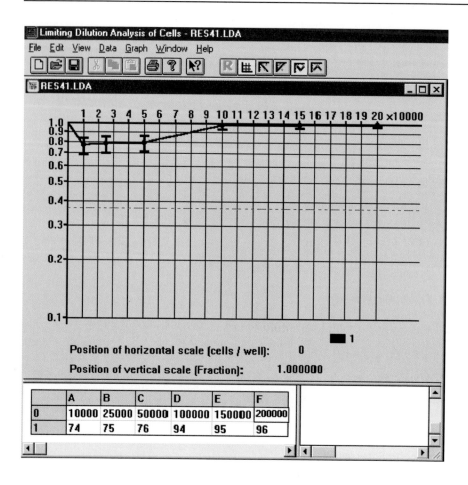

Detailed explanations are given in Chapters 6 and 7.

11.8   Advanced problems and neglected issues

11.8.1   *The number of cells in an experiment*

We have constructed the simulation so that we can account for the number of cells used to prepare each dilution. When the titration requires more cells than we have chosen, the system gives a warning. The experimenter can proceed with the titration irrespective of the warning. It is, however, suggested to chose more cells for the next experiment (i.e. more mice). The rule is: when titrating cells which are present at a very low frequency, we need a large number of cells.

11.8.2 The cell density

Dilutions are prepared from the stock cell suspension. If the user intends to use dilutions of a higher cell input than that enabled by the stock cell suspension, the simulation gives a warning which cannot be overruled (the cell input is displayed in red) (see dialog boxes of sections 11.1.4. and 11.2.4). The user has either to alter the cell input so the display is no longer red, or has to return to the earlier dialog box which asked about the source of the cells titrated (see dialog box section 11.1.2) and choose a higher cell density of the stock cell suspension. The rule is: use larger culture wells to avoid cell density problems (the Terasaki wells with a volume of 10 μl cannot be used with very high cell inputs).

11.8.3 Higher terms of Poisson distribution

Simulation provides copious information on the distribution of cells, but only the zero term of the Poisson distribution is needed for the titration plots. The reader is encouraged to use the additional information on the distribution of cells. The theoretical values of the F_1, F_2, F_3 ... terms can be compared with those obtained through simulation (see Chapter 3), and advanced LDA experiments can be constructed in which multi-hit and multi-target conditions are simulated.

11.8.4 Multi-hit and multi-target titrations

Let us assume that not only will cultures fail to respond when they lack a single precursor cell, but so will those which contain 1 precursor cell (in other words, the only cultures which respond are those containing 2 or more precursor cells). We can extract relevant data from the simulation experiment, combine F_0 and F_1 as a 'new F_0' and plot them using the LDA program.

The resulting titration curve is a 'two-hit curve' (for the theory see Chapter 5). We can set the rules as we like. In a T-cell cooperation we might want to investigate the conditions in which one B cell and at least 5 Th cells are needed for the response. All the data are there and plots can easily be constructed within the LDA program.

11.8.5 Multiplicity of Th cells

The reader should always test several different cell inputs. For example, the effect of alteration of Th-cell multiplicity on the apparent frequency of B cells can only be visualised if one performs a whole range of simulation experiments.

A typical set of results is as follows:

Table 11.4. Apparent frequency of B cells

Multiplicity of Th cells	Frequency
3	0.0000324
2	0.0000323
1	0.0000244
0.3	0.0000095
0.1	0.0000026

Note that Th multiplicity higher than '3' results in saturation (in other words, all B-cell precursors are expressed because all wells contain one or more Th-precursor cell[s]). The experiment conforms to single-hit kinetics. As soon as the multiplicity drops below '2', deviation from linearity becomes apparent, the most pronounced being at a ratio of 1 : 1.

11.8.6 Chi-square

Throughout the simulation procedure we have tacitly assumed that the linear regression line correctly represents the results. Only in the 'levelling off' experiment (section 11.5.4) have we hinted that the linear regression through the origin would be unacceptable.

'Chi-square' is a special 'quality control' feature built into the LDA program which enables us to check whether or not the linear regression line fits the data well. This feature is also available for the simulation experiments. It would have been counter-productive to interrupt the flow of the simulation procedure to instruct the reader to apply the chi-square feature.

Chi-square and its meaning is described in detail in Chapter 4, and also in the actual LDA program. If the reader has saved the results of the simulation the plots can be opened and the chi-square calculated.

11.8.7 Configurations other than Terasaki and microtitre

In section 11.1.5 the dialog box shows that there is a third option besides Terasaki and microtitre. We recommend that this system be utilised in order to explore what happens if a small number of cultures, i.e. 12 wells, are used for each dilution.

11.8.8 95% confidence limits

Readers will learn from experience about the consequences of using small numbers of cultures. They will see considerable fluctuation in the experimental outcome and the wide range of confidence limits. Plots based on 12 cultures and 120 cultures are a good start for making comparisons. The user should be aware that the highest number of cultures for calculating 95% confidence limits is 171 (the highest tabulated factorial in personal computer software is 171!).

11.8.9 Playback of the simulation

The 'remote control' for simulation has two features which we have already explored (full, short) and a third one which is explained here. Clicking on 'auto' allows us to watch all the simulation steps in slow motion, and we can interrupt the procedure in the same way as with a video recorder (VCR).

11.9 Summary

Dots are cells and cells are dots. Our intention was to *trick* the readers so that they forget that they are performing a virtual experiment, and we hope that at least in some instances they forgot the colours, grids and surfaces, and imagined B and T cells placed in microculture wells.

With the above simulation experiments, the reader can perform virtually all types of analyses which might be encountered in real experimentation. Indeed, the results of the experiments can be exported into a spreadsheet and worked on further.

What happens if we alter some of the rules of the game? For example, let's assume that negative cultures will not only be those cultures which lack the precursor cell but can also be cultures which contain one precursor cell (seeing as only cultures with 2 or more precursor cells respond). All the data are available – it is enough to merge the proper groups and open an LDA experiment (not through simulation but through the LDA program) and the data can be plotted at will. Any new rule is worth exploring. Here we refer to section 5.6 in which we deal with multi-target events. Although it is beyond the scope of these pages to deal with this additional topic, we will set up a website giving information on additional uses of the system.

Throughout most of the book we have endeavoured to ensure that each chapter could be read and followed on its own. The description on simulation is built up in a somewhat different way. The early part (B-cell titration) is explained in detail and then the reader is 'pushed' to acquire independence.

The boxes in this chapter refer to B and T cells, clones of antibody-forming cells, filler cells, soluble factors and culture conditions. They refer to the humidity in the incubator and to wrapping Terasaki trays in saran wrap. This is to give the user the illusion that the dots and screen surfaces are indeed cells and cultures.

Appendix

1   Figures from *Immunology Today*

In 1984 the authors of this monograph were asked to prepare an article on the principles of LDA for *Immunology Today* (*IT*). Judging by citations, the article was successful, and perhaps the major ingredient for its success was the colour illustrations. The figures were done in the traditional artwork procedure because computer drawing programs were not yet widely available. The centre-page colour illustrations (in two consecutive issues of *IT*, Lefkovits and Waldmann, 1984, Waldmann and Lefkovits, 1984) were the first of their kind.

The illustrations have not lost their topicality even now, 15 years later. Although we refer to the figures at several instances in this book, we have assembled them here in order to keep the colour plates in one block.

Figure A1. A single-hit curve. Four trays, each of 60 cultures, are inoculated with graded numbers of B cells (1250, 3750, 6250, 8750 cells/culture). Some of the cells in the inoculum are antigen-specific, while the majority are irrelevant third party cells. The red dots in the upper row of trays indicate the distribution of antigen-specific cells. All cells look alike and under the micro-scope the cells of interest (red dots) cannot be distinguished.

Culture conditions are chosen such that the cells of interest (red dots) have a fair chance of proliferating and after antigenic stimulation will, within a few days of culture, yield clones of daughter cells. If the original parental B cells are celled 'precursor cells', in the lower row of trays the small red dots indicate clones which develop from such precursors. Most of the companion cells in those cultures remain unaltered, some die and some others proliferate but whatever their fate they have no impact on the developing clones.

The clones produce antibody which is revealed by a haemolytic spot test or by some other assay such as ELISA or radioimmunoassay. The cultures scored positive are coloured confluent red. In the first tray of 60 cultures 24 respond, and therefore the fraction of nonresponding cultures (F_0) is 36/60 = 0.6. In the next three sets we observe that as cell input increases, the number and the proportion of negative cultures (F_0) decrease.

The results are plotted on a semi-log plot and they are expected to fit a straight line going through the origin.

Note that from the plot one can directly determine the cell input that contains an average of one precursor cell, i.e. $\mu = 1$. For $\mu = 1$, $F_0 = e^{\mu} = e^{-1} = 0.37$. Thus, by interpolating $F_0 = 0.37$, on the plot (broken line), one can read that an aliquot of 2500 cells contains 1 precursor cell. The frequency of precursor cells ($f_{prec.}$) is therefore 1/2500 or 4 x 10^{-4}. The vertical bars define the 95% confidence limits, which means that the 'true' value of F_0 is expected to fall within these interval limits in 19 out of 20 cases

Figure A2. A multi-target curve. The design of this experiment is similar to the one outlined in Figure A1 but differs in one crucial aspect: two cells are needed for expression of the clone. In the example shown a B-cell clone will only develop if both a T cell (blue) and a B cell (red) are present in a culture.

The T and B cells are assorted independently in the upper row of trays and cultures from which one or both cell types are missing will score negative for antibody; the combination of any number of T and B cells will score positive (lower rows).

The results of such an experiment follow two-target kinetics because two targets, one T cell (red) and one B cell (blue), are needed. If both kinds are present in the titrated population at a ratio of 1: 1, a curve with a definite linear portion is expected. Note that the slope is the same as for a single-hit curve. In this idealised case, however, the extrapolated straight line intercepts the *y* axis at value 2, indicating the involvement of two targets. In general, if several kinds of cells were needed for a response, a multi-target event would be expected

Figure A3. Levelling off. The general design of a limiting dilution experiment is intended to produce a straight line, in which case levelling off is undesirable. Nevertheless, levelling off is frequently observed, and can often be used to advantage as a stepping stone to uncovering the involvement of an unsuspected cell type.

The experiment depicted in this figure is a T-cell-dependent response. A positive culture is obtained if both a B cell (red) and a T cell (blue) are present in the culture. This was also true in Figure A2, but there both cell types were an integral part of the inoculum. Here a separate source of T cells is used to which B cells are admixed. In this example B cells are titrated in increasing numbers into four culture trays which contain a constant, but inadequate, number of T cells. In each tray a number of wells will contain no T cells and can thus never contribute to the generation of a B-cell clone. Thus, although the multiplicity of the B-cell population increases through the four trays the response still 'stagnates'. In other words, at higher input, where B cells are saturating, the T cells become limiting. The response levels off and asymptotically reaches an F_0 value which reflects the B-cell multiplicity. In this experiment the F_0 asymptote (broken line) is $F_0 = 0.18$; thus $F_0 = 0.18 = e^{\mu}$, and μ (the average frequency of T cells per culture) = 1.5. It is this low multiplicity of T cells (1.5) which prevents the development of B-cell clones in all cultures. To guarantee that virtually all wells acquire the required cell, the rule of thumb is to ensure that the multiplicity of μ is higher than 3 ($\mu > 3$)

Figure A4. Partition analysis. In this experiment the helper activity of (blue) T-helper cells is masked by the presence of (black) suppressive cells. Bulk culture of a mixture of T cells with B cells results in no detectable antibody response. However, at limiting input of T cells with constant numbers of B cells (red), suppressive cells (black) may be partitioned away from helper cells whose function can now be revealed. At high T-cell input the T-helper cells are present in all wells (which are for convenience shaded blue throughout). But as the cell input is further increased the suppressive cells prevail, and more and more cultures are prevented from responding

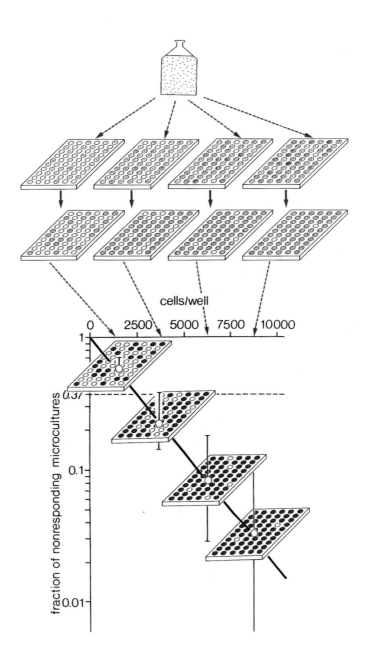

Figure A1.

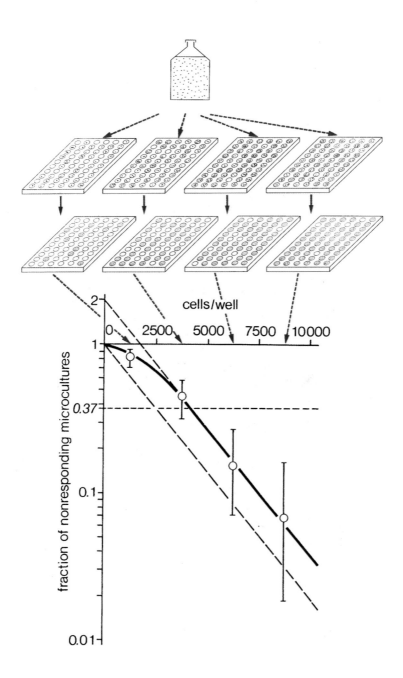

Figure A2.

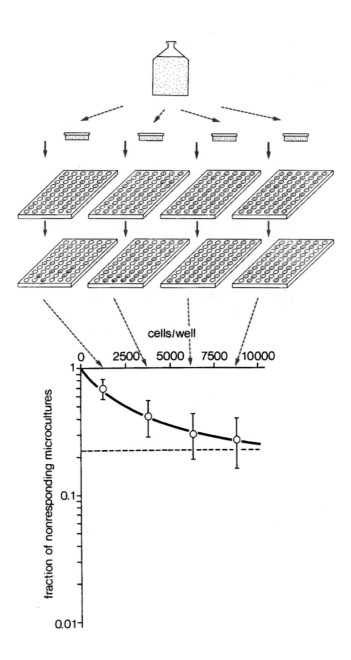

Figure A3.

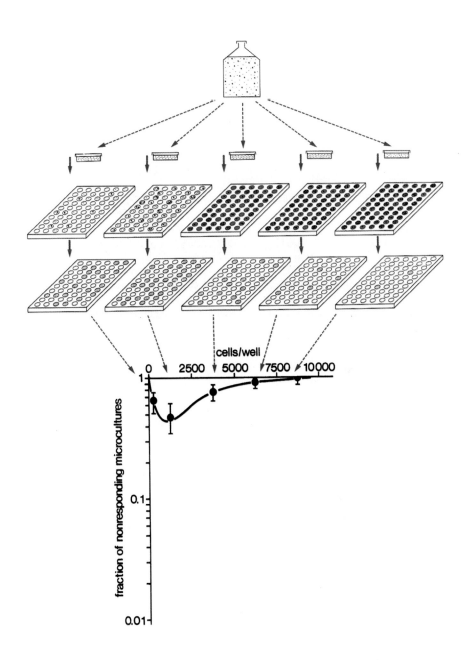

Figure A4.

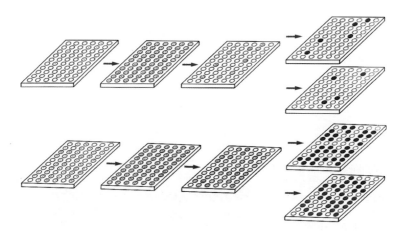

Figure A5. The monogamous T-helper cell. Evidence for contact between T and B cells in cooperation. This scheme shows a situation in which T cells have the chance of interacting with B cells of two different specificities. In the two flow sheets of the figure we consider a low or high T cell input, respectively.

In the first tray of the upper row 9 blue dots are randomly distributed in the 60 culture wells. These represent carrier-specific helper Th cell limiting dilution. To each well are added multiple B cells of two different specificities (hapten 1, red; and hapten 2, green) (tray 2). Each carrier-specific Th cell is considered fertile. On challenge with an antigen mixture (of carrier-hapten 1 or carrier-hapten 2) all wells having Th cells produce B-cell clones (tray 3), which will in turn generate antibody (upper and lower tray 4). If one Th cell could help many B cells, then many positive wells should have antibodies to both hapten 1 and hapten 2 and in the assay readout should be both green and red. In contrast, if the T cell is limited to interaction with single B cells, wells will register either green or red, but not both. It is the latter which is in fact the case.

The lower row shows the outcome of the interactions when the input of T cells is much higher: 86 carrier-specific Th cells are randomly distributed in tray 1. Monogamy still operates here but now many wells have two or more T cells, and therefore multiple B-cell clones will be activated with the appearance in many wells of two specificities of antibody (shown as red upper tray 4) and green (lower tray 4). This double antibody production simply reflects the existence of multiple T cells in individual wells

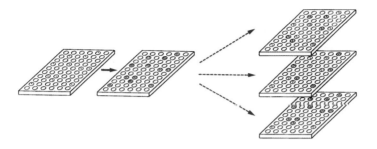

Figure A6. Multiple sampling of T-cell clones. The analysis of MHC-encoded restriction elements for T-helper cell clones. The 60 cultures of the first tray contain T cells, some of which are antigen-specific. On antigen stimulation these give rise to clones of cells (second tray). Aliquots of each clone are transferred to three plates containing antigen and B cells from three genetically different mouse strains. The subsequent development of a B-cell clone is represented by multiple red dots. The top tray contains B cells from strain A; the middle tray from strain B, and the bottom tray from (A x B)F_1. Strains A and B differ in genes of the MHC. It can be seen that members of a given T-cell clone are capable of cooperating with one but not all B-cell sources. However, they will all score positive with F_1 B cells. Note that some clones cooperate with B cells from F_1, but not from either parent

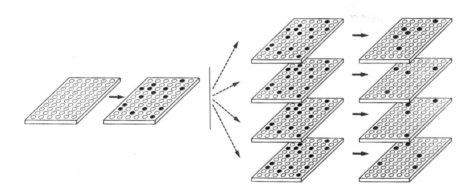

Figure A7. Heterogeneity of T-cell derived growth factors and their B cell targets. T cells stimulated with Concanavalin A produce factors which together with antigen can drive B cells to clonal proliferation. The first tray of the flow sheet shows the distribution of T cells. Only a small proportion of the cells added produce factors (blue dots), and the others are irrelevant for the analysis and therefore not displayed. The second tray shows (blue) factor production by those wells which received a suitable T cell. Aliquots of the conditioned medium (factors) are 'replica plated' onto four trays containing B cells (red dots) with antigen. What is striking is that only a fraction of the wells which receive 'factor' go on to B-cell proliferation (multiple red dots in a well) and to antibody secretion (red wells). As a control to show the presence of ample antigen-specific B cells in all wells, a pool of supernatants from individual (blue) wells will activate all 60 B-cell cultures to secretion

2 Chi-square graph

Chi-square distribution is used at several places (sections 4.3, 4.4 and 4.10) in this monograph. In all instances the calculations yield a value which is decisive for accepting or rejecting the null hypothesis. To be able to reach a decision we need to find the p value for

(i)   a given value of chi-square

(ii)   a certain number of degrees of freedom

An easy-to-use chart of χ^2 values plotted against the probability range from $p = 0.001$ to 1 was published by Bliss in 1944. The chart was reproduced in the first edition of the LDA monograph, and here we give a re-calculated and re-drawn version (prepared by Jan Rubes, co-author of the LDA software). A separate curve is drawn for each of the degrees of freedom, $df = 1$ to 30. To use the chart the reader chooses one of the 30 curves, depending on the number of degrees of freedom (indicated as df at the bottom of the chart), chooses the chi-square value on the x axis, and finds the intercept with the selected df curve. He reads the p value on the y axis. The null hypothesis (stating that there is no correlation) is accepted if the p value is larger than 0.05.

Note that the curve for 2 degrees of freedom is represented by a straight line; this is so because the chi-square distribution for 2 degrees of freedom (and only for 2 degrees of freedom) is given by an exponential function, and the graphic representation of an exponential function on a semi-log scale is a straight line.

Figure A8 (opposite page). Chi-square chart for the probability range of $p = 0.001$ to 1. A separate curve is drawn for each of the degrees of freedom, $df = 1$ to 30

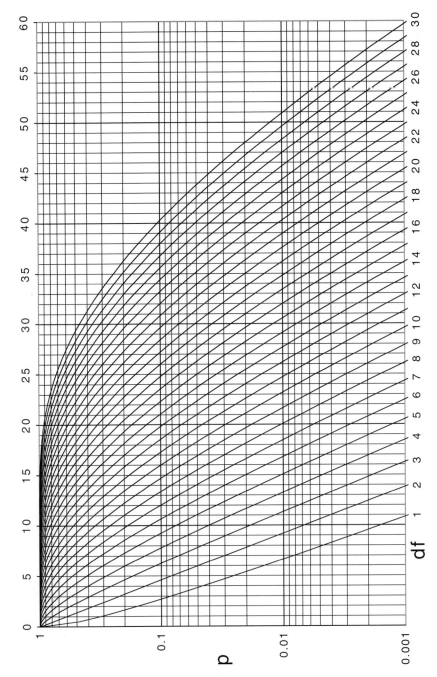

3   Tables of 95% confidence limits

The reader can obtain the values of 95% confidence limits directly from the LDA software, or alternatively look them up in one of the six tables reproduced below.

The six tables cover most of the assay configurations, i.e. Terasaki trays (60 and 120 wells per dilution) and microtitre trays (12, 24, 36 and 96 wells per dilution). A more complete set of tables can be found in Steinberg and Lefkovits (1985).

Example: in an experiment for a given cell dilution four out of 12 cultures responded.

In the table below (for $w_T = 12$) we read that four responding cultures correspond to $F_0 = 0.67$ and that the confidence limits for this fraction are 0.35 and 0.90. That is, the 'true value' of the F_0 is probably between 0.35 and 0.90, and if we assume that it is indeed in this interval, we will be wrong in only 5% of the cases.

w_R	F_0	95% confidence limits lower	upper	w_R	F_0	95% confidence limits lower	upper
0	1	0.75	– 1				
1	0.92	0.62	– 1	7	0.42	0.15	– 0.72
2	0.83	0.52	– 0.98	8	0.33	0.099	– 0.65
3	0.75	0.43	– 0.95	9	0.25	0.055	– 0.57
4	0.67	0.35	– 0.90	10	0.17	0.021	– 0.48
5	0.58	0.28	– 0.85	11	0.083	0.002	– 0.38
6	0.50	0.21	– 0.79	12	0	0	– 0.26

$w_T = 12$ (1/5 Terasaki or 1/8 microtitre trays)

		$w_T = 24$ (2/5 Terasaki or 1/4 microtitre trays)						
w_R	F_0	\multicolumn{2}{c}{95% confidence limits}	w_R	F_0	\multicolumn{2}{c}{95% confidence limits}	
		lower	upper			lower	upper
0	1	0.76 –	1				
1	0.96	0.79 –	1	13	0.46	0.26 –	0.67
2	0.92	0.73 –	0.99	14	0.42	0.22 –	0.63
3	0.88	0.68 –	0.97	15	0.38	0.19 –	0.59
4	0.83	0.63 –	0.95	16	0.33	0.16 –	0.55
5	0.79	0.58 –	0.93	17	0.29	0.126 –	0.51
6	0.75	0.53 –	0.90	18	0.25	0.098 –	0.47
7	0.71	0.49 –	0.87	19	0.21	0.071 –	0.42
8	0.67	0.45 –	0.84	20	0.17	0.047 –	0.37
9	0.63	0.41 –	0.81	21	0.125	0.027 –	0.32
10	0.58	0.37 –	0.78	22	0.083	0.010 –	0.27
11	0.54	0.33 –	0.74	23	0.042	0.001 –	0.21
12	0.50	0.29 –	0.71	24	0	0 –	0.14

		$w_T = 36$ (3/5 Terasaki or 3/8 microtitre trays)						
w_R	F_0	\multicolumn{2}{c}{95% confidence limits}	w_R	F_0	\multicolumn{2}{c}{95% confidence limits}	
		lower	upper			lower	upper
0	1	0.90 –	1				
1	0.97	0.85 –	1	19	0.47	0.30 –	0.65
2	0.94	0.81 –	0.99	20	0.44	0.28 –	0.62
3	0.92	0.78 –	0.98	21	0.42	0.26 –	0.59
4	0.89	0.74 –	0.97	22	0.39	0.23 –	0.57
5	0.86	0.71 –	0.95	23	0.36	0.21 –	0.54
6	0.83	0.67 –	0.94	24	0.33	0.19 –	0.51
7	0.81	0.64 –	0.92	25	0.31	0.16 –	0.48
8	0.78	0.61 –	0.90	26	0.28	0.14 –	0.45
9	0.75	0.58 –	0.88	27	0.25	0.121 –	0.42
10	0.72	0.55 –	0.86	28	0.22	0.101 –	0.39
11	0.69	0.52 –	0.84	29	0.19	0.082 –	0.36
12	0.67	0.49 –	0.81	30	0.16	0.064 –	0.33
13	0.64	0.46 –	0.79	31	0.14	0.047 –	0.30
14	0.61	0.43 –	0.77	32	0.111	0.031 –	0.26
15	0.58	0.41 –	0.74	33	0.083	0.018 –	0.22
16	0.56	0.38 –	0.72	34	0.056	0.007 –	0.19
17	0.53	0.35 –	0.70	35	0.028	0.001 –	0.15
18	0.50	0.33 –	0.67	36	0	0 –	0.0097

		$w_T = 60$ (1 Terasaki tray)						
w_R	F_0	95% confidence limits			w_R	F_0	95% confidence limits	
		lower		upper			lower	upper
0	1	0.94	–	1				
1	0.98	0.91	–	1	31	0.48	0.35 –	0.62
2	0.97	0.88	–	1	32	0.47	0.34 –	0.60
3	0.95	0.86	–	0.99	33	0.45	0.32 –	0.58
4	0.93	0.84	–	0.98	34	0.43	0.31 –	0.57
5	0.92	0.82	–	0.97	35	0.42	0.29 –	0.55
6	0.90	0.79	–	0.96	36	0.40	0.28 –	0.53
7	0.88	0.77	–	0.95	37	0.38	0.26 –	0.52
8	0.89	0.75	–	0.94	38	0.37	0.25 –	0.50
9	0.85	0.73	–	0.93	39	0.35	0.23 –	0.48
10	0.83	0.71	–	0.92	40	0.33	0.22 –	0.47
11	0.82	0.70	–	0.90	41	0.32	0.20 –	0.45
12	0.80	0.68	–	0.89	42	0.30	0.19 –	0.43
13	0.78	0.66	–	0.88	43	0.28	0.17 –	0.41
14	0.77	0.64	–	0.87	44	0.27	0.16 –	0.40
15	0.75	0.62	–	0.85	45	0.25	0.15 –	0.38
16	0.73	0.60	–	0.84	46	0.23	0.134 –	0.36
17	0.72	0.59	–	0.83	47	0.22	0.120 –	0.34
18	0.70	0.57	–	0.81	48	0.20	0.110 –	0.32
19	0.68	0.55	–	0.80	49	0.18	0.095 –	0.30
20	0.67	0.53	–	0.78	50	0.17	0.083 –	0.29
21	0.65	0.52	–	0.77	51	0.15	0.071 –	0.27
22	0.63	0.50	–	0.75	52	0.133	0.060 –	0.25
23	0.62	0.48	–	0.74	53	0.117	0.048 –	0.23
24	0.60	0.47	–	0.72	54	0.100	0.038 –	0.21
25	0.58	0.45	–	0.71	55	0.083	0.028 –	0.18
26	0.57	0.43	–	0.69	56	0.067	0.018 –	0.16
27	0.55	0.42	–	0.68	57	0.050	0.010 –	0.14
28	0.53	0.40	–	0.66	58	0.033	0.004 –	0.115
29	0.52	0.38	–	0.65	59	0.017	0.001 –	0.089
30	0.50	0.37	–	0.63	60	0	0 –	0.060

		$w_T = 96$ (1 microtitre tray)						

w_R	F_0	95% confidence limits			w_R	F_0	95% confidence limits		
		lower		upper			lower		upper
0	1	0.96	–	1					
1	0.99	0.94	–	1	37	0.61	0.51	–	0.71
2	0.98	0.93	–	1	38	0.60	0.50	–	0.70
3	0.97	0.91	–	0.99	39	0.59	0.49	–	0.69
4	0.96	0.90	–	0.99	40	0.58	0.48	–	0.68
5	0.95	0.88	–	0.98	41	0.57	0.47	–	0.67
6	0.94	0.87	–	0.98	42	0.56	0.46	–	0.66
7	0.93	0.86	–	0.97	43	0.55	0.45	–	0.65
8	0.92	0.84	–	0.96	44	0.54	0.44	–	0.64
9	0.91	0.83	–	0.96	45	0.53	0.43	–	0.63
10	0.90	0.82	–	0.95	46	0.52	0.42	–	0.62
11	0.89	0.80	–	0.94	47	0.51	0.41	–	0.61
12	0.88	0.79	–	0.93	48	0.50	0.40	–	0.60
13	0.86	0.78	–	0.93	49	0.49	0.39	–	0.59
14	0.85	0.77	–	0.92	50	0.48	0.38	–	0.58
15	0.84	0.76	–	0.91	51	0.47	0.37	–	0.57
16	0.83	0.74	–	0.90	52	0.46	0.36	–	0.56
17	0.82	0.73	–	0.89	53	0.45	0.35	–	0.55
18	0.81	0.72	–	0.88	54	0.44	0.34	–	0.54
19	0.80	0.71	–	0.88	55	0.43	0.33	–	0.53
20	0.79	0.70	–	0.87	56	0.42	0.32	–	0.52
21	0.78	0.69	–	0.86	57	0.41	0.31	–	0.51
22	0.77	0.67	–	0.85	58	0.40	0.30	–	0.50
23	0.76	0.66	–	0.84	59	0.39	0.29	–	0.49
24	0.75	0.65	–	0.83	60	0.38	0.28	–	0.48
25	0.74	0.64	–	0.82	61	0.36	0.27	–	0.47
26	0.73	0.63	–	0.81	62	0.35	0.26	–	0.46
27	0.72	0.62	–	0.81	63	0.34	0.25	–	0.45
28	0.71	0.61	–	0.80	64	0.33	0.24	–	0.44
29	0.70	0.60	–	0.79	65	0.32	0.23	–	0.43
30	0.69	0.58	–	0.78	66	0.31	0.22	–	0.42
31	0.68	0.57	–	0.77	67	0.30	0.21	–	0.40
32	0.67	0.56	–	0.76	68	0.29	0.20	–	0.39
33	0.66	0.55	–	0.75	69	0.28	0.19	–	0.38
34	0.65	0.54	–	0.74	70	0.27	0.19	–	0.37
35	0.64	0.53	–	0.73	71	0.26	0.18	–	0.36
36	0.63	0.52	–	0.72	72	0.25	0.17	–	0.35

cont.

cont.

		$w_T = 96$ (1 microtitre tray)					

w_R	F_0	95% confidence limits lower	upper	w_R	F_0	95% confidence limits lower	upper
73	0.24	0.16 –	0.34	85	0.115	0.059 –	0.20
74	0.23	0.15 –	0.33	86	0.104	0.051 –	0.18
75	0.22	0.14 –	0.31	87	0.094	0.044 –	0.17
76	0.21	0.13 –	0.30	88	0.083	0.037 –	0.16
77	0.20	0.124 –	0.29	89	0.073	0.030 –	0.15
78	0.19	0.115 –	0.28	90	0.063	0.023 –	0.13
79	0.18	0.107 –	0.27	91	0.052	0.017 –	0.117
80	0.17	0.098 –	0.26	92	0.042	0.011 –	0.103
81	0.16	0.090 –	0.24	93	0.031	0.007 –	0.089
82	0.15	0.082 –	0.23	94	0.021	0.003 –	0.073
83	0.14	0.074 –	0.22	95	0.010	0 –	0.057
84	0.13	0.066 –	0.21	96	0	0 –	0.038

		w_T = 120 (2 Terasaki trays)					
w_R	F_0	95% confidence limits		w_R	F_0	95% confidence limits	
		lower	upper			lower	upper
0	1	0.97 –	1				
1	0.99	0.95 –	1	37	0.69	0.60 –	0.77
2	0.98	0.94 –	1	38	0.68	0.59 –	0.76
3	0.98	0.93 –	0.99	39	0.68	0.58 –	0.76
4	0.97	0.92 –	0.99	40	0.67	0.57 –	0.75
5	0.96	0.90 –	0.99	41	0.66	0.57 –	0.74
6	0.95	0.89 –	0.98	42	0.65	0.56 –	0.73
7	0.94	0.88 –	0.98	43	0.64	0.55 –	0.73
8	0.93	0.87 –	0.97	44	0.63	0.54 –	0.72
9	0.93	0.86 –	0.97	45	0.63	0.53 –	0.71
10	0.92	0.85 –	0.96	46	0.62	0.52 –	0.70
11	0.91	0.84 –	0.95	47	0.61	0.51 –	0.70
12	0.90	0.83 –	0.95	48	0.60	0.51 –	0.69
13	0.89	0.82 –	0.94	49	0.59	0.50 –	0.68
14	0.88	0.81 –	0.93	50	0.58	0.49 –	0.67
15	0.88	0.80 –	0.93	51	0.58	0.48 –	0.66
16	0.87	0.79 –	0.92	52	0.57	0.47 –	0.66
17	0.86	0.78 –	0.92	53	0.56	0.46 –	0.65
18	0.85	0.77 –	0.91	54	0.55	0.46 –	0.64
19	0.84	0.76 –	0.90	55	0.54	0.45 –	0.63
20	0.83	0.75 –	0.89	56	0.53	0.44 –	0.62
21	0.83	0.74 –	0.89	57	0.53	0.43 –	0.62
22	0.82	0.74 –	0.88	58	0.52	0.42 –	0.61
23	0.81	0.73 –	0.87	59	0.51	0.42 –	0.60
24	0.80	0.72 –	0.87	60	0.50	0.41 –	0.59
25	0.79	0.71 –	0.86	61	0.49	0.40 –	0.58
26	0.78	0.70 –	0.85	62	0.48	0.39 –	0.58
27	0.78	0.69 –	0.85	63	0.48	0.38 –	0.57
28	0.77	0.68 –	0.84	64	0.47	0.38 –	0.56
29	0.76	0.67 –	0.83	65	0.46	0.37 –	0.55
30	0.75	0.66 –	0.82	66	0.45	0.36 –	0.54
31	0.74	0.65 –	0.82	67	0.44	0.35 –	0.54
32	0.73	0.64 –	0.81	68	0.43	0.34 –	0.53
33	0.73	0.64 –	0.80	69	0.43	0.34 –	0.52
34	0.72	0.63 –	0.79	70	0.42	0.33 –	0.51
35	0.71	0.62 –	0.79	71	0.41	0.32 –	0.50
36	0.70	0.61 –	0.78	72	0.40	0.31 –	0.49

cont.

cont.

		w_T = 120 (2 Terasaki trays)					
w_R	F_0	95% confidence limits		w_R	F_0	95% confidence limits	
		lower	upper			lower	upper
73	0.39	0.30 –	0.49	97	0.19	0.126 –	0.27
74	0.38	0.30 –	0.48	98	0.18	0.119 –	0.26
75	0.38	0.29 –	0.47	99	0.18	0.112 –	0.26
76	0.37	0.28 –	0.46	100	0.17	0.105 –	0.25
77	0.36	0.27 –	0.45	101	0.16	0.098 –	0.24
78	0.35	0.25 –	0.44	102	0.15	0.092 –	0.23
79	0.34	0.26 –	0.43	103	0.14	0.085 –	0.22
80	0.33	0.25 –	0.43	104	0.133	0.078 –	0.21
81	0.33	0.24 –	0.42	105	0.125	0.072 –	0.20
82	0.32	0.24 –	0.41	106	0.117	0.065 –	0.19
83	0.31	0.23 –	0.40	107	0.108	0.059 –	0.18
84	0.30	0.22 –	0.39	108	0.100	0.053 –	0.17
85	0.29	0.21 –	0.38	109	0.092	0.047 –	0.16
86	0.28	0.21 –	0.37	110	0.083	0.041 –	0.15
87	0.28	0.20 –	0.36	111	0.075	0.035 –	0.138
88	0.27	0.19 –	0.36	112	0.067	0.029 –	0.128
89	0.26	0.18 –	0.35	113	0.058	0.024 –	0.117
90	0.25	0.18 –	0.34	114	0.050	0.018 –	0.106
91	0.24	0.17 –	0.33	115	0.042	0.013 –	0.095
92	0.23	0.16 –	0.32	116	0.033	0.009 –	0.083
93	0.23	0.15 –	0.31	117	0.025	0.005 –	0.071
94	0.22	0.15 –	0.30	118	0.017	0.002 –	0.059
95	0.21	0.14 –	0.29	119	0.008	0 –	0.046
96	0.20	0.133 –	0.28	120	0	0 –	0.030

4   Student's *t*-test table

The use of Student's *t*-test was explained on pages 62-63 and 76-77, where also a portion of the *t*-test table was given. The table below covers the range of 1 to 30 degrees of freedom.

degrees of free-dom (df)	one tail p 0.95 0.95	two tail p 0.95 α upper 0.025 α lower 0.025	one tail p 0.99 0.99	two tail p 0.99 α upper 0.005 α lower 0.005	one tail p 0.999 0.999	two tail p 0.999 α upper 0.0005 α lower 0.0005
1	6.314	12.71	31.82	63.66	318.3	636.6
2	2.920	4.303	6.965	9.925	22.33	31.60
3	2.353	3.182	4.541	5.841	10.21	12.92
4	2.132	2.776	3.747	4.604	7.173	8.610
5	2.015	2.571	3.365	4.032	5.893	6.869
6	1.943	2.447	3.143	3.707	5.208	5.959
7	1.895	2.365	2.998	3.499	4.785	5.408
8	1.860	2.306	2.896	3.355	4.501	5.041
9	1.833	2.262	2.821	3.250	4.297	4.781
10	1.812	2.228	2.764	3.169	4.144	4.587
11	1.796	2.201	2.718	3.106	4.025	4.437
12	1.782	2.179	2.681	3.055	3.930	4.318
13	1.771	2.160	2.650	3.012	3.852	4.221
14	1.761	2.145	2.624	2.977	3.787	4.140
15	1.753	2.131	2.602	2.947	3.733	4.073
16	1.746	2.120	2.583	2.921	3.686	4.015
17	1.740	2.110	2.567	2.898	3.646	3.965
18	1.734	2.101	2.552	2.878	3.610	3.922
19	1.729	2.093	2.539	2.861	3.579	3.883
20	1.725	2.086	2.528	2.845	3.552	3.850
21	1.721	2.080	2.518	2.831	3.527	3.819
22	1.717	2.074	2.508	2.819	3.505	3.792
23	1.714	2.069	2.500	2.807	3.485	3.768
24	1.711	2.064	2.492	2.797	3.467	3.745
25	1.708	2.060	2.485	2.787	3.450	3.725
26	1.706	2.056	2.479	2.779	3.435	3.707
27	1.703	2.052	2.473	2.771	3.421	3.690
28	1.701	2.048	2.467	2.763	3.408	3.674
29	1.699	2.045	2.462	2.756	3.396	3.659
30	1.697	2.042	2.457	2.750	3.385	3.646
∞	1.645	1.960	2.326	2.576	3.090	3.291

5   Normal, *t*- and chi-square distributions

All three types of distribution belong to the category of continuous distributions. To describe such distributions we shall use the notation

$f(x)$ [read '*f* of *x*']

to denote the probability density function. Such a function is best represented by probability density curves in which the *area* under the curve is interpreted as *probability*

- the total area under the curve is 1

- the area under the curve, between x_1 and x_2 represents the probability that the continuous random variable x assumes a value between x_1 and x_2

For a small interval dx, the probability that a value of x lies in that interval is $p(x)\,dx$. In general the probability that x lies within the interval $x_1 < x < x_2$ is given by the integral

$$P(x_1 < x < x_2) \;=\; \int\limits_{x_1}^{x_2} f(x)\mathrm{d}x$$

- for a large interval x_1, x_2 the area under the curve (i.e. the probability) is large (maximal value is 1, corresponding to the total area under the curve)

- for a small interval x_1, x_2 the area under the curve (i.e., the probability) is small (note that for any single value of x the probability is zero).

Normal distribution

Normal distribution is a family of symmetric continuous distributions with two parameters

- the population mean μ, and

- the population variance σ^2

(In contrast to the *population* mean μ and *population* variance σ^2, we designate *sample* mean $\bar{x}$ and *sample* variance V.)

For the graphical representation it is convenient to use two x axis scales, as shown on the figures on the following pages

scale 1:	x	(random variable with mean μ and standard deviation σ)
scale 2:	$\dfrac{x - \mu}{\sigma}$	(determines the number of standard deviations between x and μ)

Standard normal distribution has a mean of zero and a standard deviation of 1; for this distribution the two scales are identical. Every normal distribution can be transformed by $(x - \mu)/\sigma$ into a *standard* normal distribution.

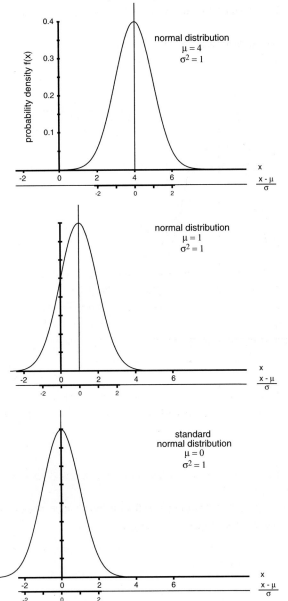

Figure A9. Normal distribution with means $\mu = 0$, 1 and 4 and variance $\sigma^2 = 1$

Three normal distributions with different means ($\mu = 4$, $\mu = 1$ and $\mu = 0$) but the same variance ($\sigma^2 = 1$) are depicted in Figure A9. The shape of the curves is the same; the third curve with $\mu = 0$ is the *standard* normal distribution.

Three normal distributions ($\mu = 0$) differing in variance ($\sigma^2 = 1$, $\sigma^2 = 2$, $\sigma^2 = 4$) are depicted in Figure A10.

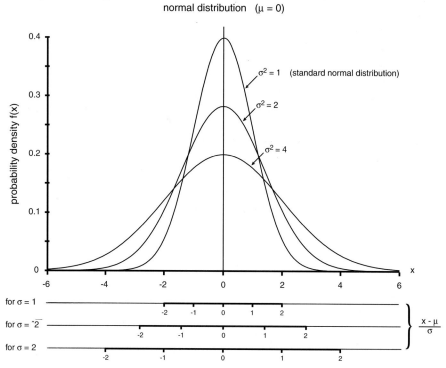

Figure A10. Normal distribution with a mean of zero but differing in variance ($\sigma^2 = 1$, 2 and 4)

The 95% rule

All normal density curves satisfy the *empirical rule* whereby 95% of the observations fall within two standard deviations of the mean, i.e. between $\mu - 2\sigma$ and $\mu + 2\sigma$.

t-*distribution*

t-distribution is a family of continuous distributions symmetric about zero having a single parameter *df* (degrees of freedom).

If *x* distributes normally (with mean μ and variance σ^2), then the *sample* mean $\bar{x}$ follows a normal distribution (with mean μ and variance σ^2/*n*, where *n* is the sample size).

If σ^2 is not known and is estimated by the *sample variance V*, then

$$t = \frac{\bar{x} - \mu}{\sqrt{V/n}}$$

is a *t*-distribution with *df* = *n* – 1, degrees of freedom.

For large *df* the *t*-distribution approaches a *standard* normal distribution. Thus, in large sample sizes we use the sample variance in place of true variance (*V* = σ^2), which for small sample sizes is not justified.

For each *n* (for each degree of freedom, *df* = *n* – 1) there is a *t*-distribution. All *t*-distributions have a mean of zero and a variance of >1. For large sample sizes (*n* > 30) the variance can be considered for all practical purposes to be equal to 1 and the *t*-distribution becomes identical to the *standard* normal distribution.

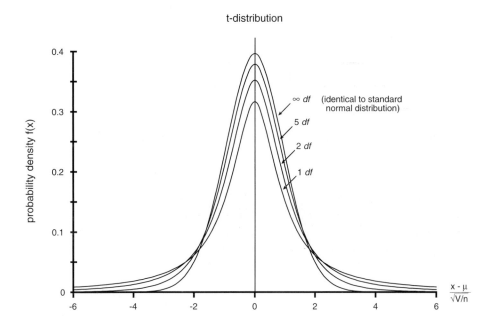

Figure A11. *t*-distributions are 'flat' for small numbers of degrees of freedom (1 *df*), and become 'taller' with increasing *df* (*df* = 2, *df* = 5). For large numbers of *df* the form of the *t*-distribution becomes identical to standard normal distribution (∞ *df*). The variance for the curve with ∞ *df* is equal to 1

Chi-square distribution

Chi-square distribution is a family of non-symmetrical (skewed) continuous distributions with a single parameter *df*, which is a positive integer.

The main use of this distribution (at least in our applications) is to determine whether the results of a particular experiment *fit* a certain probability distribution.

Definition: If random samples of size *n* are selected from a *normal* population with mean μ and variance σ², then the quantity

$$(n-1)\ \frac{V}{\sigma^2},$$

where *V* is the observed variance of the sample, and in which μ is estimated by the sample mean $\bar{x}$

is the value of a random variable having a chi-square distribution with *n* – 1 degrees of freedom.

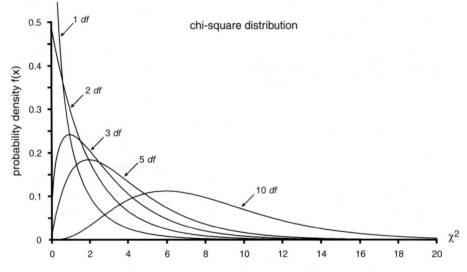

Figure A12. The chi-square distribution provides us with the description of the behaviour of the sample variance *V*. For large sample sizes the chi-square distribution is less skewed, for very large sample sizes it resembles normal distributions

6   Biographies of mathematicians

These brief biographical details of some of the mathematicians referred to in this monograph were compiled from various sources, including the *Encyclopaedia Britannica* and the *Oxford Concise Dictionary of Mathematics*.

Ernst Abbe 1840-1909
Discovered chi-square distribution in 1863.

Bernoulli

The Bernoulli family from Basle produced a stream of mathematicians, some of them very important. The best known are the brothers Jacques and Jean, and Jean's son Daniel. **Jacques Bernoulli, 1654-1705**, worked on the newly developed calculus, but is chiefly remembered for his contributions to probability theory: the *Ars conjectandi* was published after his death in 1713. He discovered the binomial distribution which is sometimes referred to as the 'Bernoulli distribution'. **Jean Bernoulli, 1667-1748**, concentrated more on calculus and was one of the founders of the *calculus of variations*. In the next generation **Daniel Bernoulli, 1700-1782**, was the member of the family whose mathematical work was mainly in the field of hydrodynamics.

Abraham De Moivre 1667-1754
English mathematician of French origin (b. Viotry, Champagne, into a French Protestant family), was one of Sir Isaac Newton's intimate friends; published *Doctrine of Chances, or Method of Calculating the Probabilities of Events at Play* which he dedicated to Newton, 1618; developed the equation describing the normal distribution, 1733, published Approximatio & Summem Terminorum Binomii (a + b) in Seriem expansi, in *Miscellans Analytica*, 1733. Later work contains the result known as *Stirling's formula* and probably the first use of the normal frequency curve.

René Descartes 1596-1650
French philosopher and mathematician who in mathematics is known mainly for his methods of applying algebra to geometry, from which analytical geometry developed. He expounded these in *La Géométrie*, in which he also used geometry to solve algebraic problems. Though named after him, Cartesian coordinates did not in fact feature in his work.

Leonhard Euler 1707-1783
The most prolific of famous mathematicians, was born in Basel, son of a Calvinist pastor from Riehen, pupil of Johannes Bernoulli but is most closely associated with the Berlin of Frederick the Great and the St. Petersburg of Catherine the Great. He worked in a highly productive period when the newly developed calculus was being extended in all directions at once, and he made contributions to most areas of mathematics, pure and applied. Among his contributions are the basic symbols, π, e and i, the summation notation Σ and the standard function notation $f(x)$. His *Introduction in analysing infinitorum* was the most important mathematics text of the late eighteenth century. In 1740 shared

a prize with Colin Maclaurin and Daniel Bernoulli 'on the tides' by the Academy of Sciences in Paris; lost his sight completely in 1766/67; completed 900 papers. Died in St. Petersburg.

Sir Ronald Aylmer Fisher 1890-1962

b. East Finchley; educated at Harrow and Cambridge, became professor of genetics 1943; knighted in 1952. His first paper (1912) introduced the method of maximum likelihood, his second dealt with the mathematical derivation of the *t*-distribution. He invented the subject of experimental design and the methods of analysis of variance and he developed the use of *contingency tables*. He continued the work of Karl Pearson (see below), writing a remarkable paper on the sampling distribution of the correlation coefficient, published in Pearson's *Biometrika* in 1915. Later a long and bitter feud with Pearson developed. As late as 1950, when a selection of his best statistical papers were published, the omission of a reference to the 1915 *Biometrika* paper was a silent reminder of the personal animosity between him and Pearson. His influential book on statistical methods appeared in 1925.

Francis Galton 1822-1911

Read his first book by the age of 3; not successful at Cambridge but received an MD from Trinity College 1840; was a first cousin to Charles Darwin: 'It may be safely declared that no one living has contributed more definitely to the progress of evolutionary study, whether by actual discovery by the fruitful direction of thought, than Mr. Galton'. In a lecture on normal distribution he used a quincunx: this is a board with nails arranged in rows in such a way that a ball placed at the start will hit a nail and will be deflected to the right and to the left. Each encounter constitutes a Bernoulli trial with $p = 0.5$. He coined the expression 'regression line', using it in his lecture on 'Regression towards mediocrity in heredity stature' at the British Association for the Advancement of Science in 1885. His best known work, published 1889, was entitled: *Natural inheritance*. He received the Darwin medal 1902.

Carl Friedrich Gauss 1777-1855

b. Braunschweig (son of a bricklayer and gardener), astronomer and mathematician, perhaps the greatest pure mathematician of all times. He was highly talented as a child. Before he was three, while watching his father's payroll calculations he detected an error and announced the correct result. There is a story that a teacher of nine-year-old Gauss told the class to work out the sum of all numbers from 1 to 100. Gauss leaned back and when reprimanded for not working on the problem, said, 'I worked it out'. The teacher said that would be impossible because just to write down the hundred numbers would take more time. Gauss replied, 'I do not need to write down the numbers because the sum of the first and the last numbers is 101, and this is also the case with the second and the last but one numbers, and as there are 50 pairs with this property, the total sum is 101 x 50 = 5050'. At the age of 11 he became acquainted with the binomial theorem. At the age of 18, he invented the method of least squares and made the new discovery that a 17-sided regular polygon could be constructed with ruler and compasses. By the age of 24, he was ready to publish his *Disquisitiones arithmeticae*. In this, he proved the *Fundamental Theorem of Arithmetic* and the *Fundamental Theorem of Algebra*. In astronomy, his great powers of mental calculation allowed him to calculate the orbits of comets and asteroids from limited observational data. He published *The Theory of the Motion of Heavenly Bodies about the Sun in Conic Sections* in 1805; one section deals with the problem of reconciling measurement error from which he deduced the form of normal distribution.

William Sealy Gosset 1876-1937

Descendant of an old Huguenot family, British industrial scientist and statistician best known for his discovery of the *t-distribution*, motivated by his research for the Guinness brewery in Dublin where he worked all his life. The most important of his papers, which were published under the pseudonym **'Student'**, appeared in 1908; described by Sir Ronald Fisher as 'Faraday of statistics'. His first mathematical paper was 'On the Error of Counting with a Haemocytometer', 1907; here he derived afresh the Poisson distribution as a limiting form of the binomial and fitted it to four series of counts of yeast cells. His next paper 'The probable error of a mean', 1908, brought him more fame for it provided the basis of Student's *t*-test.

Helmert 1875

Re-discovered chi-square distribution (after Abbe in 1863); worked out the distribution of sample variance for sampling from normal population.

Pierre Simon Laplace 1749-1827

Member of the French Royal Academy of Sciences at the age of 24, professor at the Ecole Militaire when Napoleon was a student. He derived the normal distribution independently from Gauss. In France the normal distribution is often referred to as the Laplacean distribution.

Wilhelm Lexis 1837-1914

b. Eschweiler near Aachen; graduated from the University of Bonn; research in Bunsen's chemical laboratory in Heidelberg; Strasbourg 1872; and Freiburg 1876. Bortkiewicz was his student in Bonn. He discovered that the variance between the samples will contribute relatively more to the overall variance than will the variance within the samples. When statistical values diverge from homogeneity one works with Lexis curves. This is the case when a set of balls is drawn from different urns.

Colin Maclaurin 1698-1746

Scot, who was an outstanding mathematician of the generation following Newton's. He developed and extended the subject of calculus. His textbook on the subject contains important original results, but the *Maclaurin series*, which appears in it, is just a special case of the *Taylor series* known considerably earlier. He also obtained notable results in geometry and wrote a popular textbook on algebra. He won the French Academy of Sciences prize in 1740 with Leonhard Euler and Daniel Bernoulli.

Isaac Newton 1642-1727

English physicist and mathematician, he was responsible for the law of gravity, the theory of planetary motion, the *binomial series* and Newton's method in numerical analysis. His most important published work is *Principia* (1687), the most powerful work in the history of mathematics. The unit of force, *newton*, abbreviated to 'N' is named after him. One newton is the force required to give a mass of one kilogram an acceleration of one metre per second.

Blaise Pascal 1623-1662

French mathematician noted for his work in geometry, hydrostatics and probability. Pascal's triangle, the arrangement of the binomial coefficients, was not invented by him but he did use it in his studies on probability. The unit of pressure, *pascal*, abbreviated to 'Pa' is named after him. One pascal is equal to one *newton* per square metre.

Karl Pearson 1857-1936

British statistician influential in the development of statistics for application to the biological and social sciences. Stimulated by problems in evolution and heredity, he developed fundamental concepts such as the *standard deviation*, the *coefficient of variation* and, in 1890, the *chi-squared test*. This work was contained in a series of important papers written while he was professor of applied mathematics, and then eugenics, at University College, London. He was the founder of the science of statistics and his initial statistical work was two volumes entitled, *The chances of death and other studies in evolution*. He fitted a curve to a set of observations but needed a criterion to indicate how good the fit was, and so he invented the 'chi-square' test in 1900. Asked what was the first thing he could remember, he recalled that it was sitting in a highchair and sucking his thumb. He was told to stop sucking it as it would wither away. He put his two thumbs together and looked at them for a long time. 'They look alike to me. I wonder if you would be lying to me'. This rejection of constituted authority, appeal of empirical evidence and faith in his own interpretation of the meaning of observed data were ideal attributes for following a successful path in scientific discovery. Founded the journal *Biometrika* in 1915.

Siméon Denis Poisson 1781-1840

French mathematician, born at Pithiviers, a student of J. L. Lagrange and P. S. Laplace at the Ecole Polytechnique at Paris. In 1808 he became astronomer to the 'Bureau des Longitudes', and in 1809 was appointed 'professor de la mécanique rationelle', then geometer to the Bureau des Longitudes in succession to P. S. Laplace. He was faithful to the Bourbons and after the restoration of the Bourbons, his fidelity was recognised by his elevation to the dignity of baron, though he never used the title. In 1837, he was made a peer of France. During the same year, in his paper on probability (see Chapter 2 of this monograph) he introduced the distribution that later was named after him.

Ladislaus von Bortkiewicz (also Bortkewitsch) 1868-1931

b. St. Petersburg, d. Göttingen. The work that made his name widely known was a brochure (1898) of sixty pages *Das Gesetz der kleinen Zahlen* (The law of small numbers). Poisson had shown in 1837 that besides the usual normal limit for Bernoulli's distribution there is a second limit, requiring that the number (n) of observations increases and the probability (p) decreases so that the product (np) has a limiting value. In this distribution n and p enter only through the product $\lambda = np$. Poisson's important derivation remained practically unknown for sixty years; at least, its importance was not recognised. Bortkiewicz was the first to note the fact that events in a large population, with low frequency, can be fitted by a Poisson distribution even when the probability of an event varies somewhat between the strata of the population. (The law of large numbers would be better called the law of rare events).

Frank Yates 1902-1994
Educated at Clifton College, Bristol, and Cambridge University, and is best known for the 'Yates correction for continuity' which was an improvement on the χ^2 distribution for the 2x2 table with small box values. Yates published his last paper in 1990 at the age of 88.

7   Early steps in microculture techniques

A photograph of a replicator appeared on the dust jacket of the first edition of this book. Though many laboratories still use a replicator, it gives an out-of-date impression compared to the high-tech, automatic washers, dispensers and samplers of today. In fact, it is difficult to think back to the time before this type of equipment became available and to the pre-replicator days.

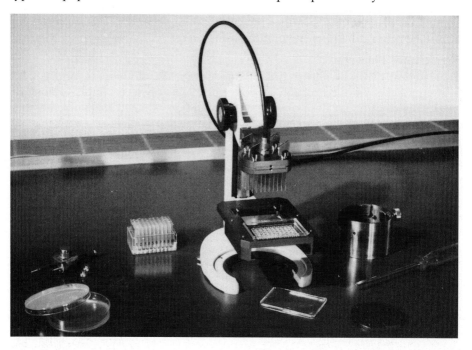

Figure A13. Replicator

The first experiments which led to the development of LDA were devised a few weeks after the conclusion of an EMBO course held in November 1967 at the Paul Ehrlich Institute, Frankfurt, Germany. Niels Jerne, director of the Institute, organised an immunology course entitled 'On plaques and rosettes'. At this course Dick Dutton introduced a new method for inducing antibody responses *in vitro*. When the course was over, a group of scientists (Claudia Henry, Hiroshi Fuji and Ivan Lefkovits – one of the authors of this monograph) inherited the leftovers, including the Dutton medium (later correctly referred to as *Mishell–Dutton* medium), feeding cocktails, rocker platforms, plexiglas incubation boxes and the working batch of sheep red blood cells.

Ivan Lefkovits decided to carry out a fluctuation test which was well known in a different context from papers by Luria and Delbrück (1943). The miniaturisation of the Mishell–Dutton technique was not straightforward because no microplates for cell cultures were available. Although 96-well plates for performing haemolytic or haemagglutination tests existed, they were toxic for the cultures. Once it was recognised that neither suitable plastic nor glassware were available, the hunt for finding a nontoxic microculture support was on. After trial and error, successful cultures were grown on Parafilm sheets (yes, they already existed). With a sterile glass rod we punched dimples into sterile Parafilm (only rarely did we have any contamination). Cell suspensions with added antigen were pipetted with Falcon plastics pipettes (with tips pulled under heat). The Parafilm wells with varying volumes of cell suspension (10 to 20 µl) were covered with a sheet of Parafilm, bent at the edge to seal the wells. Incubation was performed in plexiglas boxes, similar to those used today. The Mishell–Dutton protocol required 'daily feeding' of the cultures so we had to provide the microcultures with the nutrients, and this was done by spraying the Parafilm layer with feeding cocktail using a sterile perfume flacon.

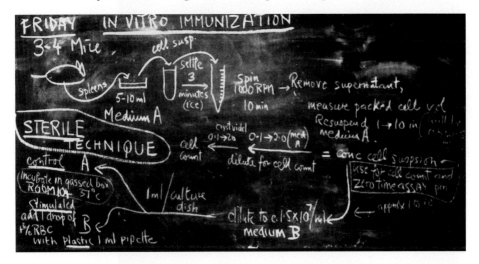

Figure A14. Photograph of the blackboard on which Dick Dutton described the experimental protocol for the *in vitro* immune response

At the end of the incubation period the Parafilm array was cut into individual wells, and these were immersed in tubes containing BSS. The content was vortexed briefly and the empty Parafilm well retrieved and discarded with forceps. The cells were washed and plated to detect plaque-forming cells. The whole content of the tube was plated. Once we saw that the culture medium at the end of the culture period contained enough antibody to lyse a layer of red cells, we developed a spot test. Using a thin-tipped Falcon plastic pipette we released a sample from the Parafilm well onto a Petri dish containing a layer of red cells. After the droplet had soaked in, we added complement and incubated it for about 30 minutes. Zones of lyses indicated positive cultures.

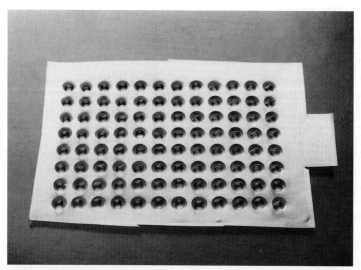

Figure A15 Culture wells (dimples) punched with a sterile glass rod into Parafilm sheets

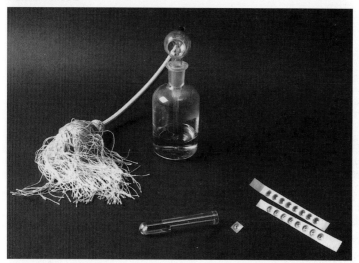

Figure A16. Perfume flacon with 'nutritional cocktail' was used for spraying the Parafilm cultures with feeding cocktail

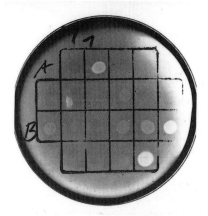

Figure A17. Spot test on red cells embedded in agar. Zones of lysis (droplets of culture medium soaked in the SRBC-agar layer plus complement) indicate the presence of anti-SRBC antibody

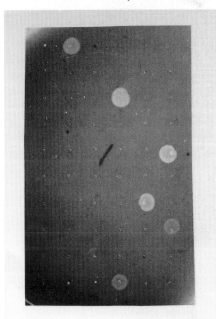
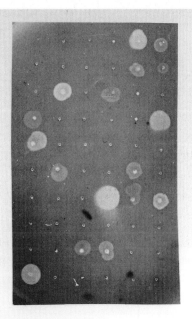

Figure A18. Spot test as performed with the replicator

8   Pascal's triangle

Pascal's triangle is an arrangement of numbers consisting of n rows, each having one more number than the previous one, and the numbers obey the following rules:

- the zero row contains only the number 1, while all the other rows start with number 1 and end with number 1

- every number in the triangle is equal to the sum of the two numbers which are situated above it to the left and right (the number 3 in row 3 is the sum of $1 + 2$, the number 21 in row 7 is the sum of $6 + 15$)

- the sum of the numbers in each row equals to 2^n

- the numbers in the triangle represent the coefficients of the expression $(a + b)^n$:

  thus, for row 6, the numbers 1, 6, 15, 20, 15, 6, 1, correspond to:

  $$(a+b)^6 = a^6 + 6a^5b + 15a^4b^2 + 20a^3b^3 + 15a^2b^4 + 6ab^5 + b^6$$

Pascal's triangle

n	triangle expansion	2^n
0	1	1
1	1 1	2
2	1 2 1	4
3	1 3 3 1	8
4	1 4 6 4 1	16
5	1 5 10 10 5 1	32
6	1 6 15 20 15 6 1	64
7	1 7 21 35 35 21 7 1	128
8	1 8 28 56 70 56 28 8 1	256

- there are additional rules and symmetries about the numbers along the sides of the triangle, e.g. 1, 2 ,3, 4, 5, 6 or 1, 3, 6, 10, 15, 21 (in the latter set, the difference between the neighbouring numbers is 2, 3, 4, 5, 6 . . .)

and we conclude the list of rules by stating the most important rule that

- each row represents the binomial coefficient $\binom{n}{r}$ where n is the row number and $r = 0, 1, \ldots, n$.

Note that the formula for the binomial coefficient is:

$$\binom{n}{r} = \frac{n(n-1)\times\ldots\times(n-r+1)}{1\times 2\times\ldots\times r} = \frac{n!}{r!(n-r)!}$$

Row 6 can be written as:

$$\binom{6}{r} = \frac{6!}{r!(6-r)!} = 1, \ 6, \ 15, \ 20, \ 15, \ 6, \ 1$$

The binomial coefficients on p. 52 (section 4.4) are those of row 8 of Pascal's triangle.

Pascal's triangle and probability

If we divide the numbers of any given row with the number in the right margin (2^n) we obtain fractions, as exemplified (again) by row 6:

$$\frac{1}{61}, \ \frac{6}{64}, \ \frac{15}{64}, \ \frac{20}{64}, \ \frac{15}{64}, \ \frac{6}{64}, \ \frac{1}{64}$$

also

$$\frac{1}{64} + \frac{6}{64} + \frac{15}{64} + \frac{20}{64} + \frac{15}{64} + \frac{6}{64} + \frac{1}{64} = 1$$

$$0.015625 + 0.09375 + 0.234375 + 0.3125 + 0.234375 + 0.09375 + 0.015625 = 1$$

The numbers represent probabilities of the binomial distribution in 'draws with replacement'.

The properties of Pascal's triangle can be visualised by a quincunx test (see next Appendix section).

9   Quincunx

An apparatus to test the p values of the binomial distribution is called a quincunx. Nails or pins are arranged in a simple way to enable a ball (e.g. a metal
ball-bearing) to go through the horizontal gaps between the nails. The nails in
successive rows are placed centrally to the gaps of the previous row. A set of
balls is placed at the start and allowed to fall. As the balls descend they
encounter the nails and have an equal chance of being diverted to the right or
to the left. Each encounter constitutes a Bernoulli trial with $p = 0.5$. The con-
tainers at the bottom of the quincunx serve to count the outcome of the trials.
Binomial distribution with other than $p = 0.5$ can be simulated by tilting the
quincunx so that there is a bias to one direction.

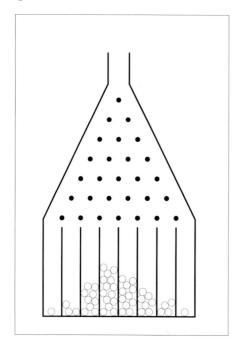 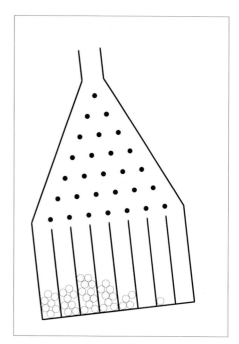

Figure A19. Quincunx. An apparatus to test the p values of the binomial distribution. The con-
tainers at the bottom serve to count the outcome of the trials. The tilted quincunx simulates
binomial distributions in which we expect other values of p than $p = 0.5$

10 Cartesian coordinates and quadrants

In the Cartesian coordinate system the axes divide the plane into four regions called quadrants. By convention the numbering is as follows:

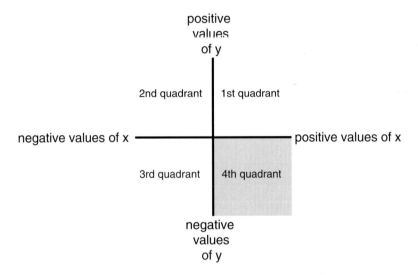

positive values of y

2nd quadrant | 1st quadrant

negative values of x ——————— positive values of x

3rd quadrant | 4th quadrant

negative values of y

LDA graphical representation is confined to the 4th quadrant. The word 'Cartesian' originates from the name René Descartes.

Positive and negative slope: linear equations ($y = ax$, $y = ax + b$) have positive or negative values of a, and the lines point upwards or downwards.

Linear equations and graphs for lines through the origin:

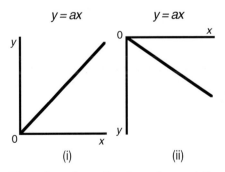

$y = ax$ $y = ax$

(i)   (ii)

The value a is positive for a slope pointing upwards (i) and negative when pointing downwards (ii)

Linear equations and graphs for lines not passing through the origin:

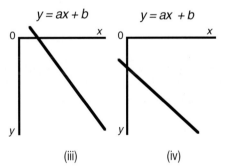

$y = ax + b$ $y = ax + b$

(iii)   (iv)

The value b is positive in the left-hand graph (iii), negative in the right-hand one (iv)

11   Molecular components of a lymphocyte

The mass of an adult mouse is about 20 g. The spleen of such a mouse weighs about one percent of the whole animal, i.e. 200 mg. Most of the cells in a spleen are lymphocytes – about 1-2 x 10^8 per spleen.

The resting cells possess a different set of molecules than the blast cells do. Change to effector cells (plasma cells as antibody-producing 'end' cells and various forms of helper and cytotoxic cells) results in further change of the molecular components (see also Lefkovits, 1995).

Composition and mass of a lymphocyte (mass in Daltons)

	Resting cell (diameter 7 μm volume 180 μm³)	Blast cell (diameter 11 μm volume 700 μm³)	Plasma cell (diameter 16 μm volume 2150 μm³)
Chromosomes	8 x 10^{12}	8 x 10^{12}	8 x 10^{12}
Ribosomes in the nucleolus	2 x 10^{12}	1 x 10^{13}	1.4 x 10^{13}
RNA	4 x 10^{11}	2 x 10^{12}	3 x 10^{12}
Nuclear envelope	2 x 10^{11}	4 x 10^{11}	6.8 x 10^{11}
Water	3.8 x 10^{13}	4 x 10^{13}	2.0 x 10^{13}
Nucleus	**4.86 x 10^{13}**	**6.04 x 10^{13}**	**4.57 x 10^{13}**
Endoplasmic reticulum and Golgi	4 x 10^{12}	5 x 10^{13}	40 x 10^{13}
Mitochondria	2 x 10^{13}	10 x 10^{13}	20 x 10^{13}
Lysosomes Endosomes Secretory granules	-	6 x 10^{12}	1.5 x 10^{13}
Cytoskeleton	1 x 10^{12}	5 x 10^{12}	2 x 10^{13}
Cytosol	2.6 x 10^{13}	17.3 x 10^{13}	51.7 x 10^{13}
Membrane	8 x 10^{11}	1.6 x 10^{12}	2.4 x 10^{12}
Cytoplasm and membrane	**5.18 x 10^{13}**	**33.6 x 10^{13}**	**115.4 x 10^{13}**
Total mass (i.e. nucleus, cytoplasm and membrane)	**1 x 10^{14}**	**4 x 10^{14}**	**1.2 x 10^{15}**

For comparison the mass of organelles (in Daltons) and some other complex structures are given:

1 chromosome	1.7 x 10^{11}	1 lysosome	1.3 x 10^{10}
DNA of 1 chromosome	1 x 10^{11}	1 nuclear pore	1 x 10^8
1 mitochondrion	1 x 10^{11}	1 ribosome	4.5 x 10^6

The mass of the DNA in a chromosome is roughly equal to the mass of 1 mitochondrion, which in turn is about the mass of an *E. coli* bacterium.

12   List of equations

[The numbers in brackets refer to the page numbers on which the equations appear.]

Constants, logarithms, limits

$$\ln_e e - 1 \qquad [24]$$

$$e^\mu = \frac{\mu^0}{0!} + \frac{\mu^1}{1!} + \frac{\mu^2}{2!} + \frac{\mu^3}{3!} + \frac{\mu^4}{4!} + \cdots \qquad [25]$$

$$\lim_{x \to \infty}\left(1 - \frac{1}{x}\right) = 1 \qquad [25]$$

$$\lim_{x \to \infty}\left(1 - \frac{1}{x}\right)^x = e^{-1} \qquad [25]$$

$$\lim_{w \to \infty}\left(1 - \frac{1}{w}\right)^c = e^{-\frac{c}{w}} \qquad [26]$$

Mean, variance, standard deviation

$$V = \frac{\Sigma\,(r - \mu)^2}{w} \qquad [23, 24]$$

$$\sigma = \sqrt{V} = \sqrt{\frac{\Sigma\,(r - \mu)^2}{w}} \qquad [23]$$

$$\mu = \frac{\Sigma\,r}{w} = \frac{c}{w} \qquad [24]$$

$$\Sigma\,(r - \mu) = 0 \qquad [24]$$

$$\text{mean} = \Sigma r F_r \qquad [30]$$

Probability

$$p = \frac{1}{w} \qquad [17]$$

$$q = 1 - \frac{1}{w} \qquad [17]$$

$$p + q = 1 \qquad [17]$$

Binomial

$$P_r = \frac{c!}{r!\,(c - r)!}\, p^r\, q^{c-r} \qquad [17]$$

$$P_r = \binom{c}{r}\, p^r\, q^{c-r} \qquad [20]$$

$$\binom{c}{r} = \frac{c!}{r!\,(c - r)!} \qquad [20]$$

Poisson

$$F_0 = e^{-\mu} \qquad [27]$$

$$F_r = \frac{\mu^r}{r!}\, e^{-\mu} \qquad [29]$$

$$\ln F_0 = \ln e^{-\mu} \qquad [32]$$

$$\mu = -\ln F_0 \qquad [32]$$

$$F_0 = 1 - \left(1 - e^{-\mu}\right)^m \qquad [87]$$

$$F_0 = 1 - \left(1 - e^{-\mu_B}\right)\left(1 - e^{-\mu_T}\right) \qquad [88]$$

$$F_0 = e^{-\mu_B} + e^{-a\mu_B} - e^{-(a+1)\mu_B} \qquad [88]$$

$$F_0 = e^{-\mu_B} + e^{-\mu_T} - e^{-(\mu_B + \mu_T)} \qquad [89]$$

$$F_0 = 1 - e^{-\mu_{Ts}} + e^{-(\mu_{Th} + \mu_{Ts})} \qquad [95]$$

Poisson *(cont.)*

$$F_0 = \left(1 + \mu + \frac{\mu^2}{2} + \cdots + \frac{\mu^{n-1}}{(n-1)!}\right)e^{-\mu}$$

[86]

$$\frac{\mathrm{d}F_0}{\mathrm{d}\mu_{Th}} = \frac{1}{R}e^{-\frac{1}{R}\mu_{Th}} - \frac{R+1}{R}e^{-\frac{R+1}{R}\mu_{Th}}$$

[97]

$$F_0 = 1 - \left(1 + \mu_{Ts} + \frac{\mu_{Ts}^2}{2} + \ldots + \frac{\mu_{Ts}^{a-1}}{(a-1!)}\right)\left(1 - e^{-\mu_{Th}}\right)e^{-\mu_{Ts}}$$

[98]

Slope

$$a_{upper} = a + t_{\frac{\alpha}{2}, n-1}\sqrt{\frac{1}{n-1}\left(\frac{\Sigma y_i^2}{\Sigma x_i^2} - a^2\right)}$$

$$a_{lower} = a - t_{\frac{\alpha}{2}, n-1}\sqrt{\frac{1}{n-1}\left(\frac{\Sigma y_i^2}{\Sigma x_i^2} - a^2\right)}$$

[60]

$$a_{upper} = a + t_{\frac{\alpha}{2}, n-2}\sqrt{\frac{\frac{1}{n-2}\Sigma(y_i - \hat{y}_i)^2}{\Sigma x_i^2 - \frac{1}{n}(\Sigma x_i)^2}}$$

$$a_{lower} = a - t_{\frac{\alpha}{2}, n-2}\sqrt{\frac{\frac{1}{n-2}\Sigma(y_i - \hat{y}_i)^2}{\Sigma x_i^2 - \frac{1}{n}(\Sigma x_i)^2}}$$

[61]

$$b_{upper} = b + t_{\frac{\alpha}{2}, n-2}\sqrt{\left(\frac{1}{n-2}\Sigma(y_i - \hat{y}_i)^2\right)\left(\frac{1}{n} + \frac{\left(x - \frac{1}{n}\Sigma x_i\right)^2}{\Sigma x_i^2 - \frac{1}{n}(\Sigma x_i)^2}\right)}$$

[61]

$$b_{lower} = b - t_{\frac{\alpha}{2}, n-2}\sqrt{\left(\frac{1}{n-2}\Sigma(y_i - \hat{y}_i)^2\right)\left(\frac{1}{n} + \frac{\left(x - \frac{1}{n}\Sigma x_i\right)^2}{\Sigma x_i^2 - \frac{1}{n}(\Sigma x_i)^2}\right)}$$

[61]

References

Arienti, F., J. Sule-Suso, C. Melani, C. Maccalli, F. Belli, M. T. Illeni, A. Anichini, N. Cascinelli, M. P. Colombo, G. Parmiani. 1994. Interleukin-2 gene-transduced human melanoma cells efficiently stimulate MHC-unrestricted and MHC-restricted autologous lymphocytes. *Hum. Gene Ther.* 5: 1139-1150

Bateman, H. 1910. On the probability distribution of α particles. *Phil. Mag.* 20: 704-707

Batten, P., T. Heaton, S. Fuller-Espie, R. I. Lechler. 1995. Human anti-mouse xenorecognition. Provision of noncognate interactions reveals plasticity of T cell repertoire. *J. Immunol.* 155: 1057-1065

Berkson, J. 1980. Minimum chi-square, not maximum likelihood! *Ann. Stat.* 8: 457-487

Bieganowska, K. D., L. J. Ausubel, Y. Modabber, E. Slovik, W. Messersmith, D. A. Hafler. 1997. Direct ex vivo analysis of activated, Fas-sensitive autoreactive T cells in human autoimmune disease. *J. Exp. Med.* 185: 1585-1594

Blau, M., K. Altenburger. 1922. Ueber einige Wirkungen von Strahlen II. *Z. Physik.* 12: 315-326

Bliss, C. I. 1944. A chart of the chi-square distribution. *J. Am. Stat. Assoc.* 39: 246-248

Bortkewitsch, L. see von Bortkewitsch, L

Brod, S. A., D. Benjamin, D. A. Hafler. 1991. Restricted T cell expression of IL-2/IFN-gamma mRNA in human inflammatory disease. *J. Immunol.* 147: 810-815

Bunjes, D., M. Theobald, B. Hertenstein, M. Wiesneth, J. Novotny, R. Arnold, H. Heimpel. 1995a. Successful therapy with donor buffy coat transfusions in patients with relapsed chronic myeloid leukemia after bone marrow transplantation is associated with high frequencies of host-reactive interleukin 2- secreting T helper cells. *Bone Marrow Transplant.* 15: 713-719

Bunjes, D., M. Theobald, T. Nierle, R. Arnold, H. Heimpel. 1995b. Presence of host-specific interleukin 2-secreting T helper cell precursors correlates closely with active primary and secondary chronic graft-versus-host disease. *Bone Marrow Transplant.* 15: 727-732

Burnet, F. M. 1957. A modification of Jerne's theory of antibody production using the concept of clonal selection. *Aust. J. Sci.* 20: 67-68

Campbell, G. A. 1923. Probability curves showing Poisson's exponential summation. *Bell System Techn. J.* 2: 95-112

Chen, W. F., A. Wilson, R. Scollay, K. Shortman. 1982. Limiting dilution assay and clonal expansion of all T cells capable of proliferation. *J. Immunol. Methods.* 52: 305-314

Chou, Y. K., D. N. Bourdette, H. Offner, R. Whitham, R. Y. Wang, G. A. Hashim, A. A. Vandenbark. 1992. Frequency of T cells specific for myelin basic protein and myelin proteolipid protein in blood and cerebrospinal fluid in multiple sclerosis. *J. Neuroimmunol.* 38: 105-113

Clarke, R. D. 1946. An application of the Poisson distribution. *J. Inst. Actuaries.* 72: 481

Clopper, C. J., E. S. Pearson. 1934. The use of confidence on fiducial limits illustrated in the case of the binomial. *Biometrika.* 26: 404-413

Corley, R. B., B. Kindred, I. Lefkovits. 1978. Positive and negative allogeneic effects mediated by MLR-primed lymphocytes. Quantitation by limiting dilution analysis. *J. Immunol.* 121: 1082-1089

Crowther, J. A. 1924. Some considerations relative to the action of x-rays on tissue cells. *Proc. Roy. Soc.* B96: 207-214

Desaymard, C., H. Waldmann. 1976. Evidence for the inactivation of precursor B cells in high dose unresponsiveness. *Nature.* 264: 780-782

Dessauer, F. 1922. Ueber einige Wirkungen von Strahlen I. *Z. Physik.* 12: 38-47

Dorling, A., G. Lombardi, R. Binns, R. I. Lechler. 1996. Detection of primary direct and indirect human anti-porcine T cell responses using a porcine dendritic cell population. *Eur. J. Immunol.* 26: 1378-1387

Dozmorov, I. M., V. V. Kalinichenko, I. A. Sidorov, R. A. Miller. 1995a. Antagonistic interactions among T cell subsets of old mice revealed by limiting dilution analysis. *J. Immunol.* 154: 4283-4293

Dozmorov, I., V. Kalinichenko, G. Suss, K. Shortman. 1995b. Regulatory cellular interactions in the primary mixed lymphocyte reaction. *Immunol. Letters.* 46: 43-48

Dozmorov, I. M., R. A. Miller. 1996. Regulatory interactions between virgin and memory CD4 T lymphocytes. *Cell. Immunol.* 172: 141-148

Dozmorov, I. M., G. V. Lutsenko, I. A. Sidorov, R. A. Miller. 1996. Analysis of cellular interactions in limiting dilution cultures. *J. Immunol. Meth.* 189: 183-196

Eisenhart, C., P. W. Wilson. 1943. Statistical methods and control in bacteriology. *Bacteriological Reviews.* 7: 57-137

Fazekas de St. Groth, S. 1982. The evaluation of limiting dilution assays. *J. Immunol. Meth.* 49: R11-R23

Feld, B. T., G. Szilard. 1972. *The collected works of Leo Szilard*: MIT Press

Finney, D. J. 1951. The estimation of bacterial densities from dilution series. *J. Hyg.* 49: 26-35

Finney, D. J. 1964. *Statistical method in biological assay.* 2nd ed. London: Charles Griffin & Co. Ltd.

Fisher, R. A. 1915. Frequency-distribution of the values of the correlation coefficient in samples from an indefinitely large population. *Biometrika.* 10: 507-511

Fisher, R. A. 1925. *Statistical methods for research workers.* Edinburgh: Oliver & Boyd

Gordon, R. D. 1939. Estimating bacterial populations by the dilution methods. *Biometrika*. 31: 167-180

Gowans, J. L., D. D. McGregor. 1963. The origin of antibody-forming cells. In *Immunopathology, IIIrd International Symposium*, eds. P. Grabar, P. A. Miescher, 89-92. Basel: Schwabe

Haldane, J. B. S. 1939. The mean and variance of χ^2, when used as a test of homogeneity, when expectations are small. *Biometrika*. 31: 346-355

Hayward, A. R., G. O. Zerbe, M. J. Levin. 1994. Clinical application of responder cell frequency estimates with four years of follow up. *J. Immunol. Methods*. 170: 27-36

He, X. S., H. S. Chen, K. Chu, M. Rivkina, W. S. Robinson. 1996. Costimulatory protein B7-1 enhances the cytotoxic T cell response and antibody response to hepatitis B surface antigen. *Proc. Natl. Acad. Sci. U.S.A.* 93: 7274-7278

Hornick, P. I., P. A. Brookes, P. D. Mason, K. M. Taylor, M. H. Yacoub, M. L. Rose, R. Batchelor, R. I. Lechler. 1997. Optimizing a limiting dilution culture system for quantifying the frequency of interleukin-2-producing alloreactive T helper lymphocytes. *Transplantation*. 64: 472-479

Hünig, T., A. Schimpl, E. Wecker. 1974. Autoradiographic studies on the proliferation of antibody-producing cells *in vitro*. *J. Exp. Med*. 139: 754-760

Jerne, N. K. 1955. The natural selection theory of antibody formation. *Proc. Natl. Acad. Sci. USA*. 41: 849-857

Jerne, N. K., A. A. Nordin, C. Henry. 1963. The agar plaque technique for recognizing antibody-producing cells. In *Cell-Bound Antibodies*, eds. B. Amos, H. Koprowski, 109-125. Philadelphia: Wistar Institute Press

Jerne, N. K. 1967. Summary: Waiting for the end. *Cold Spring Harbor Symposia on Quantitative Biology*. 23: 591-603

Julius, M. H., E. Simpson, L. A. Herzenberg. 1973. A rapid method for the isolation of functional thymus-derived murine lymphocytes. *Eur. J. Immunol*. 3: 645-649

Keever, C. A., M. Abu-Hajir, W. Graf, P. McFadden, P. Prichard, J. O'Brien, N. Flomenberg. 1995. Characterization of the alloreactivity and anti-leukemia reactivity of cord blood mononuclear cells. *Bone Marrow Transplant*. 15: 407-419

Lefkovits, I. 1972. Induction of antibody-forming cell clones in microcultures. *Eur. J. Immunol*. 2: 360-365

Lefkovits, I., O. Kamber. 1972. A replicator for handling and sampling microcultures in tissue culture trays. *Eur. J. Immmunol*. 2: 365-366

Lefkovits, I., J. Quintans, A. Munro, H. Waldmann. 1975. T-cell dependent mediator and B-cell clones. *Immunology*. 28: 1149-1154

Lefkovits, I., H. Waldmann. 1977a. B cell subsets in nude mice. In *Proceedings of the 2nd International Workshop on Nude Mice*, eds. T. Nomura, N. Ohsawa, N. Tamaoki, K. Fujiwara, 171-183. Tokyo: Tokyo Press

Lefkovits, I., H. Waldmann. 1977b. Heterogeneity of B cells reacting with T cell factors. Evidence for matching T cell and B cell subsets. *Immunology.* 32: 915-922

Lefkovits, I., H. Waldmann. 1984. Limiting dilution analysis of the cells of immune system. I. The clonal basis of the immune response. *Immunol. Today.* 5: 265-268

Lefkovits, I., J. R. Frey, C. Coleclough. 1995. Human lymphocyte cDNA ordered library analyzed by 2D gel electrophoresis II. Frequency distribution of mRNA populations. *Appl. Theor. Electrophoresis.* 5: 43-47

Lefkovits, I. 1995. . . . And such are little lymphocytes made of. *Res. Immunol.* 146: 5-10

Li, Y., W. P. Stefura, F. E. Simons, F. T. Jay, K. T. HayGlass. 1994. Limiting dilution analysis of antigen stimulated IL-4 and IFN-gamma production in human mononuclear cell populations. *J. Immunol. Methods.* 175: 169-179

Li, Y., F. E. Simons, F. T. Jay, K. T. HayGlass. 1996. Allergen-driven limiting dilution analysis of human IL-4 and IFN-gamma production in allergic rhinitis and clinically tolerant individuals. *Int. Immunol.* 8: 897-904

Lindahl, K. F., D. B. Wilson. 1977. Histocompatible antigen activated cytotoxic T lymphocytes. II. Estimates of the frequency and specificity of precursors. *J. Exp. Med.* 145: 508-521

Lister, J. 1878. On the nature of fermentation. *Quarterly J. Microscop. Sci.* 18: 177-194

Lucas, K. G., T. N. Small, G. Heller, B. Dupont, R. J. O'Reilly. 1996. The development of cellular immunity to Epstein-Barr virus after allogeneic bone marrow transplantation. *Blood.* 87: 2594-2603

Luria, S. E., M. Delbrück. 1943. Mutations of bacteria from virus sensitivity to virus resistance. *Genetics.* 28: 491-511

Marrack, P., J. W. Kappler. 1975. Antigen-specific and non-specific mediators of T cell/B cell cooperation. I. Evidence for their production by different T cells. *J. Immunol.* 114: 1116-1125

Mason, P. D., C. M. Robinson, R. I. Lechler. 1996. Detection of donor-specific hyporesponsiveness following late failure of human renal allografts. *Kidney Int.* 50: 1019-1025

Mather, K. 1949. The analysis of extinction time data in bioassay. *Biometrics.* 5: 127-143

Matuszewski, T., J. Neyman, J. Supinska. 1936. Über die Wahrscheinlichkeit der Reinkulturisolierung aus einer Petrischale. *Zentr. Bakt. Parasitenk.* 95: 45-53

McFarland, E. J., P. A. Harding, D. Luckey, B. Conway, R. K. Young, D. R. Kuritzkes. 1994. High frequency of Gag- and envelope-specific cytotoxic T lymphocyte precursors in children with vertically acquired human immunodeficiency virus type 1 infection. *J. Infect. Dis.* 170: 766-774

Miller, J. F. A. P. 1960. Studies on mouse leukemia. The role of the thymus in leukaemogenesis by cell free leukaemic filtrates. *Brit. J. Cancer.* 14: 93-99

Miller, J. F. A. P., N. L. Warner. 1971. The immune response of normal, irradiated and thymectomized mice to fowl immunoglobulin-G as detected by a hemolytic plaque technique. *Int. Arch. Allergy.* 40: 59-71

Mishell, R. I., R. W. Dutton. 1967. Immunization of dissociated spleen cell cultures from normal mice. *J. Exp. Med.* 126: 432-442

Molina, E. C., R. P. Crowell. 1924. Deviation of random samples from average conditions and significance to traffic men. *Bell System Tech. J.* 3: 88-89

Montagna, D., R. Maccario, P. Comoli, L. Prete, M. Zecca, E. Giraldi, C. Daielli, A. Moretta, P. De Stefano, F. Locatelli. 1996. Frequency of donor cytotoxic T cell precursors does not correlate with occurrence of acute graft-versus-host disease in children transplanted using unrelated donors. *J. Clin. Immunol.* 16: 107-114

Nelder, J. A., R. W. M. Wedderburn. 1972. Generalized linear models. *J. R. Statist. Soc.* 135: 370-384

Neyman, J. 1941. Fiducial argument and the theory of confidence intervals. *Biometrika.* 32: 128-150

Pearson, K. 1924. Historical note on the origin of the normal curve of errors. *Biometrika.* 16: 402-404

Pearson, E. S. 1939. Note on the inverse and direct methods of estimation in R. D. Gordon's problem. *Biometrika.* 31: 181-186

Pearson, E. S., H. O. Hartley. 1958. *Biometrika tables for statisticians.* 2nd ed, Vol. 1. Cambridge: Cambridge University Press

Phillips, J. M., H. Waldmann. 1977. Monogamous T helper cell. *Nature (Lond.).* 268: 641-642

Poisson, S. D. 1837. *Recherches sur la Probabilité des Jugements en Matière Criminelle et en Matière Civile, précédées des Règles Générales du Calcul des Probabilités.* Paris: Bachelier

Rittenberg, M. B., A. A. Amkraut. 1966. Immunogenicity of trinitrophenyl-haemocyanin: production of primary and secondary anti-hapten precipitins. *J. Immunol.* 97: 421-430

Rosenkrantz, K., C. Keever, K. Bhimani, A. Horvath, J. Brochstein, R. O'Reilly, B. Dupont, N. Flomenberg. 1990. Both ongoing suppression and clonal elimination contribute to graft- host tolerance after transplantation of HLA mismatched T cell-depleted marrow for severe combined immunodeficiency. *J. Immunol.* 144: 1721-1728

Rutherford, E., H. Geiger. 1910. The probability variations in the distribution of α particles. *Phil. Mag.* 20: 698-704

Satyanarayana, K., Y. K. Chou, D. Bourdette, R. Whitham, G. A. Hashim, H. Offner, A. A. Vandenbark. 1993. Epitope specificity and V gene expression of cerebrospinal fluid T cells specific for intact versus cryptic epitopes of myelin basic protein. *J. Neuroimmunol.* 44: 57-67

Schreier, M. H., A. A. Nordin. 1977. An evaluation of the immune response *in vitro*. In *B and T cells in immune recognition*, eds. F. Loor, G. E. Roelants, 127-152. Chichester: J. Wiley and Sons

Schrödinger, R. 1944. *What is life?* Cambridge: Cambridge University Press

Schwarer, A. P., Y. Z. Jiang, P. A. Brookes, A. J. Barrett, J. R. Batchelor, J. M. Goldman, R. I. Lechler. 1993. Frequency of anti-recipient alloreactive helper T-cell precursors in donor blood and graft-versus-host disease after HLA-identical sibling bone-marrow transplantation. *Lancet*. 341: 203-205

Schwarer, A. P., Y. Z. Jiang, S. Deacock, P. A. Brookes, A. J. Barrett, J. M. Goldman, J. R. Batchelor, R. I. Lechler. 1994. Comparison of helper and cytotoxic antirecipient T cell frequencies in unrelated bone marrow transplantation. *Transplantation*. 58: 1198-1203

Skinner, M. A., J. Marbrook. 1976. An estimation of the frequency of precursor cells which generate cytotoxic lymphocytes. *J. exp. Med.* 143: 1562-1567

Steinberg, C., T. Lefkovits. 1985. Tables for evaluating limiting dilution experiments. In *Immunological Methods*, eds. I. Lefkovits, B. Pernis, vol. 3, 317-373. Orlando: Academic Press

Stinissen, P., C. Vandevyver, R. Medaer, L. Vandegaer, J. Nies, L. Tuyls, D. A. Hafler, J. Raus, J. Zhang. 1995. Increased frequency of gamma delta T cells in cerebrospinal fluid and peripheral blood of patients with multiple sclerosis. Reactivity, cytotoxicity, and T cell receptor V gene rearrangements. *J. Immunol.* 154: 4883-4894

Student. 1907. On the error of counting with a haemocytometer. *Biometrika*. 5: 351-360

Student. 1908. The probable error of a mean. *Biometrika*. 6: 1-25

Taswell, C. 1981. Limiting dilution assays for the determination of immunocompetent cell frequencies. I. Data analysis. *J. Immunol.* 126: 1614-1619

Taswell, C. 1987. Limiting dilution assays for the separation, characterization, and quantitation of biologically active particles and their clonal progeny. In *Cell Separation: Methods and Selected Applications*, eds. T. G. Pretlow II, T. P. Pretlow, vol. 4, 109-145. Orlando: Academic Press

Teh, H.-H., E. Harley, R. A. Phillips, R. G. Miller. 1977. Quantitative studies on the precursors of cytotoxic lymphocytes. I. Characterization of a clonal assay and determination of the size of clones derived from single precursors. *J. Immunol.* 118: 1049-1056

Thorndike, F. 1926. Applications of Poisson's probability summation. *Bell System Techn. J.* 5: 604-624

van Oers, M. H., J. Pinkster, W. P. Zeijlemaker. 1978. Quantification of antigen-reactive cells among human T lymphocytes. *Eur. J. Immunol.* 8: 477-484

van Oers, M. H., J. Pinkster, W. P. Zeijlemaker. 1979. Cooperative effects in mitogen- and antigen-induced responses of human peripheral blood lymphocyte subpopulations. *Int. Arch. Allergy Appl. Immunol.* 58: 53-66

von Bortkewitsch, L. 1898. *Das Gesetz der kleinen Zahlen*. Leipzig: Verlag B. G. Teubner

Waldmann, H., I. Lefkovits, J. Quintans. 1975. Limiting dilution analysis of helper T-cell function. *Immunology*. 28: 1135-1148

Waldmann, H., I. Lefkovits, A. Feinstein. 1976a. Restriction in the functions of single helper T cells. *Immunology*. 31: 353-362

Waldmann, H., P. Poulton, C. Desaymard. 1976b. Antigen nonspecific factor in B cell activation. Origin, biological properties and failure to show a relationship to H-2. *Immunology*. 30: 723-733

Waldmann, H., H. Pope. 1977. Can B cell tolerance be generated by oligovalent thymus dependent antigens? *Immunology*. 32: 657-667

Waldmann, H., G. Kenny, A. Feinstein, B. Brown. 1978. The monogamous T helper cell. In *Proc. 12th Leuk. Culture Conference*, 111-116. New York: Academic Press

Waldmann, H., I. Lefkovits. 1984. Limiting dilution analysis of the cells of immune system. II. What can be learnt? *Immunol. Today*. 5: 295-298

Welch, B. L. 1937. The significance of the difference between two means when the population variances are unequal. *Biometrika*. 29: 350-362

Zhang, Y., M. Cosyns, M. J. Levin, A. R. Hayward. 1994. Cytokine production in varicella zoster virus-stimulated limiting dilution lymphocyte cultures. *Clin. Exp. Immunol*. 98: 128-133

Zimmer, K. G. 1961. *Studies on Quantitative Radiation Biology*. Edinburgh: Oliver and Boyd, Ltd.

Index

Table and figure page numbers are set in italics
Computer program commands are set in bold

Limiting Dilution Analysis

DATE _____

EXPERIMENT _____

cells/well

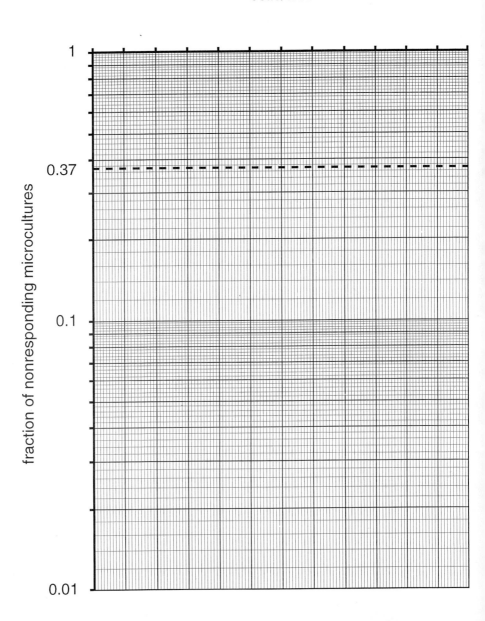

Installation note for the LDA software: LDA Grapher (evaluation of experiments)
LDA Simulation (simulation program)
2×2 table calculator
LDA Help (help file for LDA Grapher)
web links
data-example files

Installation requirements: IBM Personal Computer or 100 percent compatible with an
80386 or higher processor
RAM 16 MB or more
Hard disk drive with at least 4MB free space
Mouse
Floppy disk drive 3.5 inch
Windows 95 or Windows NT 4.0 operating system

Installation procedure:
1. Insert the floppy disk #1 into the drive
2. Press **Start**, choose **Run** and type [A]:\setup.exe where [A] is the floppy
drive identifier (A or B)
3. Follow the onscreen instructions

Step 1 - Setup
Options: [x]   Install products
             [ ]   Uninstall products
Select the first choice and press **Next**

Step 2 - Operating system
Options: [x]   Install 32 bit applications (short directory names convention)
             [ ]   Install 32 bit applications (long directory names convention)
Select the first choice (default) and press **Next**

Step 3 - Setup
Options: [x]   Typical
             [ ]   Minimal
             [ ]   Custom
Select the first choice (default) and press **Next**

Step 4 - Selection of the products to install
Options: [x]   LDA software package
Click the checkbox on the left side and press **Next**

Step 5 - Confirmation of the update of duplicate files
Options: [x]   Prompt for each
             [ ]   Overwrite all
             [ ]   Overwrite none
             [ ]   Rename existing
             [ ]   Alternate directory
If you are installing the software first time, select the first choice. If you are re–installing the
software, select the second choice. Then press **Next**

Step 6 - Install products (the installer will request insertion of disk 2)
Options: [x]   Install now
             [ ]   Exit
Select the first choice and press **Next**

Step 7 - Installation ready
To finish installation press **Finish**

Technical notes and support via e-mail::
http://www.path.ox.ac.uk/lda
poisson@bohem-net.cz